I0409607

Prologue

CR Hornbeck-Kaiser is a CPA and educator with three earned degrees (including a Masters) who taught Business, Math and Computer Science classes for Denver Technical College (now DeVry University).

This book explains how to lose overweight and obese pounds without dieting and then how to maintain that weight loss. Best of all the desired result is achieved while continually feasting on truly delicious foods. As a result hunger is eliminated.

The "1 to 5 Weight Loss Without Dieting" book (Aptly subtitled: "Guide to the Low-Carb Regimen") is unique in its approach. In simple steps with menus, references and recipes this book shows the reader how to achieve the much sought after goal of simply and easily losing weight.

Most important of all, the book explains how a properly applied low-carb regimen is foundational to overcoming insulin resistance, a precursor to adult onset diabetes as well as certain forms of heart disease and cancer.

Further, the book demonstrates that a properly adopted low-carb regimen may be the key to overcoming the epidemic of excess weight and obesity that affects two thirds of our nation.

TABLE OF CONTENTS

—

RECIPES

Chapter One

Introduction to the LCR

The Low-Carb Regimen (LCR) is not a diet: We do not diet, we feast up to eight times per day on the most amazingly delicious foods! (See the **Sample Menu**.)

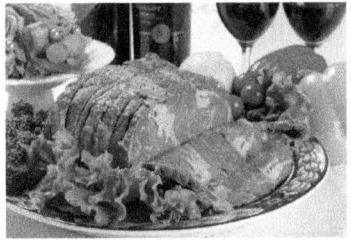 This is my kind of a regimen: Losing weight and gaining healthful vitality by never being truly hungry as a result of constantly eating the right kinds of flavourful, nutritious low-carb foods!

I. Losing weight without dieting:

You are probably reading this book because you are looking for an easy, effective and efficient way to lose weight.

Good news: For the majority of those seeking to lose weight, this approach is easy, effective and efficient! Frankly, it is by far the easiest, most effective and most efficient weight-loss method I have ever encountered.

A KEY To Success: Unlike other methods, we eliminate hunger.

- Unlike other methods, we maintain our weight loss.

- Unlike other methods, we address the pre-diabetic condition (insulin resistance) that may ultimately impact over half of our population.

A GAME CHANGER: Insulin resistance may be the key factor (along with our national tendency to consume increasing quantities of highly refined high carb foods) in our nation's epidemic of obesity. There is much more to tell you but (since this is the internet generation where we are used to getting what we want in seven seconds or less):

II. Here's how it works:

1. You will overcome your highly refined, high carb addiction.

What? You didn't know you were addicted to highly refined, high carb foods? If you are a typical American, you are addicted. You'll have to read on to learn more about this! (By the way: Don't panic – overcoming an addiction to highly refined, high carb foods is relatively simple!)

2. You will consume adequate nourishment each day.

Many of the foods in the typical American diet have questionable nutritional value. See **Chapter Ten** for ideas on food supplementation. In particular, those eating "low-carb" should consider Vitamin D-3.

3. You will activate your fat-burning metabolism.

What? You didn't know you had a fat-burning metabolism? (You thought you only had a "fat accumulating" metabolism!) You'll have to read on to learn more about this!

4. You will optimize your fat-burning metabolism.

Think of the effort involved in losing weight as being like the fuel you put in your car. You want to get all the mileage you can out of that fuel. Similarly, you'll want to optimize the weight-loss benefits of the effort you put into your fat-burning metabolism.

5. You will ultimately include previously excluded foods.

Surely you do not want to live the rest of your life on only the lowest carb foods? There is much to know about the amazing nutrition and weight-loss maintenance that comes from selected higher carb foods.

6. You will maintain your weight-loss and increased vitality for a lifetime

None of us wants to be one of those individuals who loses 65 pounds and then gains back two or three times as much. You'll have to read on to learn more about avoiding this pitfall!

Note: The remainder of this chapter lays the groundwork for The Five Steps of the Low-Carb Regimen along with the related focal points that support our weight-loss without dieting experience. The information that follows can greatly aid in your success in the LCR. For those who do not wish to understand the precepts and the limitations of the Low-Carb Regimen, you may wish to:

- Go directly to Chapter Three: **Step One –** Overcoming Carb Withdrawal

- Go directly to the **Cooking Guide** located at the back of this book

On the other hand, if you (like me!) would like to understand why you are doing what you are doing and what works and does not work, please read the rest of this chapter (Chapter One) and continue through Chapter Two before beginning "Step One – Overcoming Carb Withdrawal" (Chapter Three).

III. Reading this book:

Alright! We've established that deciding to read this book may help you in your pursuit. Since you want to lose weight easily, efficiently and effectively, you need the knowledge that enables you to understand:

- how this is achieved and

- how you can make it work in your own experience.

Note: A wonderful paraphrase applies here. The paraphrase states that "without knowledge people perish." Let me apply this to my personal experience. When it came to my personal failure in my numerous prior weight-loss efforts, my previous lack of knowledge regarding the LCR proved my undoing. If only I had known how easy it is to truly lose weight (once our fat-burning metabolism activates, the fat is eliminated as our bodies convert the fat into energy)! With the proper knowledge I could have kept myself from needless frustration and the sense of guilt over my failure. In those days I thought to myself, "Other people seem to be able to mange their weight – why can't I find the weight-loss success that I seek?"

IV. Most find success:

Most who learn how to implement the LCR and who follow its precepts, lose weight, increase vitality and – best of all – maintain their weight loss. This statement follows from research published in the Journal for the American Medical Association in which low-carb dieting is demonstrated to be an effective weight-loss approach for most participants.

"Wait a minute!" you say. "Just MOST?"

1. "What about ME?" you ask.

Disclaimer time: If you are an individual with an underlying health condition that interferes with your ability to safely activate a fat-burning metabolism through a properly followed LCR, then – of course –

you are not most people. Individuals in this category are encouraged to seek the guidance and counsel of their qualified health-care professionals.

It is expected, however, that most are able to respond well to a properly followed Low-Carb Regimen. If you are like most people, then this approach holds the potential to produce beneficial results.

2. "What about strenuous workouts?" you ask.

A pattern of ongoing strenuous exercise normally calls for sufficient carbohydrate input to fuel the demands created by the heavy-impact activities undertaken. Distance runners and other endurance athletes will NOT want to undertake the LCR. Further, strenuous exercise interferes with a fat-burning metabolism, and a fat-burning metabolism is key to effective Low-Carb Regimen weight-loss.

a) Light Aerobic Exercise

On the other hand, light aerobic exercise – for instance a relaxing 10 to 20 minute walk (up to three times daily) – tends to support the fat-burning metabolism created by the LCR.

The amazing thing in all this is that it is not necessary to exercise strenuously in order to lose weight IF you have established a fat-burning metabolism (Again, strenuous exercise is actually counterproductive to the LCR!).

b) Weight-Loss Without Strenuous Exercise

Rather than exercise strenuously in an effort to lose weight, we simply change what we eat to conform to the Five Steps of the LCR and – once we activate a fat-burning metabolism – our overweight pounds from excess fat tend to take care of themselves. When I first encountered this amazing truth, I was skeptical. After all, it only seemed "right" that there should be serious pain and suffering for the dietary indiscretions that created my rotund self. Surely I would not lose weight unless I sweated and agonized in some kind of rigorous workout and starvation process?

c) Counterproductive Weight-Loss Dependencies

In fairness to the strain generated by gym workouts, there can be a certain amount of camaraderie with our fellow sufferers. Fellowship benefits aside, let me emphasize, again, this LCR truth: Those who thrive on the camaraderie that occurs in strenuous workouts at the gymnasium may find that their "need" for heavy duty workouts is counterproductive to the LCR weight-loss without dieting creation of a fat-burning metabolism.

A companion danger for fans of strenuous workouts is that they may be tempted to participate in celebrations that obviously undermine the LCR weight-loss without dieting. For instance, most of us know someone whose participation in the "gym social structure" also involves the weekly "Hey, it's Friday – we've earned the right to party!" carbaholic binging.

3. "What about our weight-loss expectations?" you ask.

It is reasonable to expect that the average individual – after allowing for their gender, body-frame, and age – could achieve a non-overweight status per the BMI (Body Mass Index) scale.

This does not mean, however, that all men will achieve the body-frame of the latest "hunk" male movie star, or that all women will attain the figure of a super model.

I can tell you from personal experience that the sixty-five pounds of weight-loss needed to move me from the obese to the overweight and then to the non-overweight categories of the Body Mass Index have created a dramatic improvement in my appearance. However, although I look remarkably better and can now wear much more flattering clothes, no one would ever mistake me for a movie star!

On the other hand, I feel like a "star" on a daily basis with my improved health, vitality, energy level, sense of well-being and much more active lifestyle.

4. "What about the rate at which we lose weight?" you ask.

A potential reason for chronic obesity is insulin resistance. Switching to a properly followed low-carb regimen can aid in dealing with this pre-diabetic condition. After all, excessive body fat – especially belly fat – is frequently associated with insulin resistance.

Accordingly, the typical low-carb weight-loss experience is that the obese pounds shed more easily. A slower weight-loss rate, then, is often experienced for the top half of the overweight range (one step below "obese") while the last ten pounds that lead to the upper limit of one's ideal weight tend to shed most slowly of all. In spite of different rates of weight loss for the various levels of our excess pounds, arrival at the upper level of our ideal weight is a reasonable expectation.

V. Why you should try this:

With the ideas above in place, here are a few key reasons why you should give the Low-Carb Regimen serious consideration as a means for losing weight and increasing vitality.

- **First,** nothing else you've tried has worked. You either haven't lost weight or you have gained back weight after you lost it. You may even have added to the pounds with which you started.

- **Second,** successful use of the Low-Carb Regimen is well documented in scientific and popular literature. Here are some quick references (much more is available throughout this book):

1. Kekwick and Pawain in the 1950s and 60s

. . . researched low-carb, high fat and high protein dieting. They identified a *FMS* (fat-mobilizing substance) that appeared in the urine of people whose metabolisms were successfully burning body fat. When this substance was injected into mice, it stimulated the fat burning process in the test animals. Kekwick and Pawain's work influenced many researching the field of weight gain and obesity.

2. A subsequent study explored the work of Dr. Alfred W. Pennington

. . . who recommended removing all starch and sugar from meals. An article exploring Pennington's work, titled "A New Concept in the Treatment of Obesity", was published in the October 1963 issue of the **Journal of the American Medical Association** by Edgar S. Gordon, Marshall Goldberg, and Grace J. Chosy, and advocated the complete elimination of sugar from the diet and a marked increase in both fat and protein. This work influenced and was adopted by Dr. Robert Atkins who sought a solution to his own personal struggle with weight gain.

3. In 1972 Dr. Robert Atkins

. . . popularized low-carb, high fat and high protein dieting in his book, "Dr. Atkins Diet Revolution." Additional publications and popularity came through the work of The Atkins Center. Atkins revised and republished his original book in 1992. Both of his editions were best sellers.

4. Decades of research

. . . established insulin resistance (also, see the detailed references in **Chapter Fifteen** of this book) as a link to diabetes, hypertension, certain forms of heart disease, certain forms of cancer and various other diseases. Weight gains resulting in subjects becoming overweight and/or obese correlate highly – but not always – with insulin resistance. A common visible result of insulin resistance is the tendency to accumulate body fat, particularly around the belly. Failure to adequately deal with insulin resistance makes weight loss difficult.

5. In the 1990s and continuing through today

. . . the Journal of the American Medical Association (JAMA) began to publish studies verifying the effectiveness of a low-carb regimen as a means of weight loss.

6. In 2011, Dr. Paul Magarelli

. . . began free seminars in the Colorado Springs area. Although I gratefully attended several of the seminars, I did not become a patient of the good doctor nor did I become a participant in his program. Instead, I began my own research on the low-carb regimen and applied the concepts gained from all of the above referenced sources into my own LCR.

7. By the end of 2012 your author lost sixty-five pounds

. . . over a period of twelve months by following the LCR detailed in this book. In addition, your author achieved this by never going hungry, by feasting on the most wonderful meals he can ever recall eating and by doing this up to eight times per day. The weight-loss gains and vitality increases continue into 2013 (and beyond!). Your author – having journalized the experience throughout – publishes this book with the desire to inspire and aid others who struggle with weight loss.

No one seeking to lose weight should have to go through what I experienced before adopting the LCR. Everyone seeking to lose weight should have the opportunity to benefit from the simple and easy weight loss that is possible through the LCR.

I see people who struggle with weight loss all around me (two thirds of our population is either obese or overweight). Many have given up. One could only wish those who are overweight could know how easy it is to lose weight.

The desire to communicate this amazing truth, frankly, has become the "magnificent obsession" that requires this book.

Third, (my testimonial) the LCR is the only weight-loss plan that has worked for me. Over the years I lost 104 pounds and gained back 190: Other approaches that I have used – calorie counting, weight loss pills, dietary drinks, exercising, fad diets, etc. – left me feeling hungry, tired, sore and with only temporary (if any) results. I could NOT maintain the unrealistic and ineffective methods of these approaches. Worst of all was the ongoing discomfort of hunger. On the other hand, now I no longer feel hungry. In the LCR you eat before (or, at the very least, when) you feel hungry.

Fourth, you could experience the following benefits:

1. The LCR provides the potential

for reducing the cost of groceries purchased. Over time – as we lose weight – it takes less food to make us full, and this can reduce our grocery bill. Although results depend on your meal selections, in my experience groceries cost less now than when I was sixty-five pounds heavier!

2. The LCR tends to increase

health and vitality. In my own experience, the "two to four sinus infections per year" that plagued me throughout my adult life are now a thing of the past. After all, excess weight is a drag on the immune system and a harbinger of potential disease to come.

3. Less sick time and increased energy can result

in increased drive, motivation, and productivity, and – applied properly – this can increase your potential for success in life.

4. For the majority of people, the LCR is

not only easy, efficient and effective, but in addition it can eliminate the excess cost of hiring health-care professionals to manage your weight-loss for you (a mega-million dollar industry in America).

5. Properly achieved weight-loss tends to promote

self-esteem and confidence which in turn can positively impact your life. The list of potential benefits could go on and on, but you get the idea!

VI. The insulin resistant

As noted earlier in this chapter, the LCR appears to be particularly helpful for those of us who are insulin resistant. This makes sense since those of us in this category have an affinity for taking carbohydrates and converting them into fat cells. To put it mildly, we are really good at packing fat on our bods!

1. An Epidemic of Overweight and Obese Americans

You may or may not be in this category (nearly two thirds of our adult population are). On the other hand, the developing epidemic of obesity in America (whose roots some trace back to the dietary and lifestyle changes over the last one hundred years or so), gives evidence that something has gone wrong in our nutritional approach.

2. An Introduction to Insulin Resistance (see Chapter Fifteen for more detailed information)

Our American food culture is inundated with breads, potatoes, pastas, starches, and sugar-rich foods. These are all carbohydrates and many are highly-refined high carb foods.

Our bodies are designed to convert carbohydrates into glucose for use as energy in our cells. The glucose must be transported to our cells and our bodies produce insulin for this purpose.

a) CGI Metabolism and Carbaholism

Although the carbohydrate-glucose-insulin (CGI) metabolism is a marvel of biochemical engineering, it can "break down" under the "weight" of a constant barrage of too many carbs habitually eaten over time.

Keep in mind that "carbaholism" (my term by which I mean the ongoing over-consumption of carbohydrates) has become a national pastime in America.

In this situation, our cells begin to "resist" the insulin transporting the over-abundance of glucose and we become insulin resistant (a pre-diabetic state and a foreshadower of numerous minor to major health issues). The excess glucose (from too many carbohydrates) that our cells now reject ultimately becomes stored as fat and we end up looking like inverted light bulbs.

b) The Insulin Capable Versus The Insulin Resistant

On the other hand, perpetually thin over-eaters – instead of being insulin resistant – may be excessively insulin "capable." By this I mean, that their metabolisms – instead of struggling to process carbohydrates – may be extremely efficient in this process. As a result, they appear to be able to eat whatever they want without storing excess fat.

As noted before the insulin resistant, are much too "efficient" at converting carbohydrate to fat. As a result, we are the ones who are likely to survive longer when in a starvation situation because, potentially, we can survive on our stored fat!

From this viewpoint, insulin resistance might be a blessing in disguise though most of us trying to overcome our overweight conditions would not see it this way.

Accordingly, those who are insulin resistant may need to cut back on carbohydrates and increase protein, low-carb dairy (cheese, butter and cream), low-carb vegetables (avoid starchy vegetables like potatoes and carrots), and low-carb fruits (berries and melons) in their diet in order to reduce excess fat on their bodies.

In other words, the insulin resistant get (need) to replace the nourishment depleted non-foods of our fast food commerce with delicious, nutritious REAL food! (If you are still craving that chocolate cake, you have my sympathy – but there are much better, tastier, more satisfying, more nutritious and more healthful options!)

VII. The Glycemic Index:

We've mentioned it, but what is it?

The glycemic index was included by Dr. Robert C. Atkins, author of **Dr. Atkins New Diet Revolution** and founder of the **Atkins diet**, as a useful means for food selection.

According to Wikipedia: The glycemic index, glycaemic index, or GI is a measure of the effects of carbohydrates in food on blood sugar levels. It estimates how much each gram of available carbohydrate (total carbohydrate minus fiber) in a food raises a person's blood glucose level following consumption of the food, relative to consumption of glucose. Glucose has a glycemic index of 100, by definition, and other foods have a lower glycemic index.

1. Glycemic Index and the Carbohydrate-Glucose-Insulin (CGI) Metabolism

The **glycemic index** was promoted by Dr. Atkins in order to help his patients in their low-carb dieting efforts.

a) Carbohydrates Are Glucose Waiting To Happen

This makes better sense when you keep in mind (as described above) that our bodies are designed to convert carbohydrates into glucose (blood sugar) in the bloodstream. To review, our bodies then produce

---

insulin in order to transport the glucose to our cells for absorption and use as cell energy. This process creates a relatively "immediate" energy supply for our cells.

b) The Idea Behind The Glycemic Index

Highly refined carbohydrates (essentially processed and, in some cases, concentrated carbs) become in our bodies like glucose on steroids: They are rapidly absorbed and processed in our metabolisms and they create dramatic blood-sugar spikes.

The idea of the glycemic index, then, is to identify foods that are particularly "good" at spiking our blood sugar (so that we might avoid them).

Conversely, foods that are "low" on the glycemic index are supposed to be alright. I want to offer caution on this assumption:

My wife and I recently encountered a spaghetti product that is supposed to be "low glycemic." This product emphasizes on its packaging that it has 5 grams of digestible fibers. On the other hand, the required FDA food labeling indicated that a single serving of this product contained 41 grams of carbs with virtually no fiber. Needless to say, we did not buy this product.

As we seek to eat low-carb, we need to keep in mind that fiber is just one of three sub-categories of carbohydrate. Most fiber is non-digestible and, therefore, is subtracted from total carb count (see the section in Chapter Two on **Grasping Net Carb Count**).

c) Keeping It Simple

At first all of this can seem a bit confusing.

To keep it simple, I have found it more than sufficient to simply keep my net carb count below 50 net grams of carbs per day. With no disrespect intended for those who religiously follow it, the glycemic index is an interesting, but – for me – unnecessary concept in the early steps of the LCR: I simply eat following the LCR as described in this book and weight and related concerns take care of themselves!

A little homage, now, to a former geography teacher and football coach: The coach always told us to keep it simple: Just tackle the guy with the ball. In the same way, I encourage readers to keep their low-carb quest simple: Eat the foods that are low in net carbs per the Low-Carb Regimen.

2. Then: A Personal Experience

Just before I began eating according to the concepts in the LCR, I tipped the scale in my doctor's office at 244 pounds and was wearing a pair of pants with a 46 to 48 inch waist span. I am only five foot, ten and one half inches tall and for my body frame 202 pounds is obese while between 182 pounds and 201 pounds is overweight. See the following table for more information on overweight and obese ranges: **Body Mass Index Table**.

I knew that just being overweight dramatically increased the likelihood of a host of ailments as well as a shortened and diminished lifespan.

I was concerned, but being like most Americans in this situation, I "blew off" my concerns, took my prescriptions for my sinus infections (the reason I had gone to the doctor in the first place) and, while I was at Safeway picking up that prescription, made certain that I got a couple of more loaves of ciabatta bread. (I felt lousy and I just "knew" the bread would make me feel better. After all, there was still some room left in those 48 inch waist pants . . .)

3. Now: A Personal Experience

Today, I'm sitting in the cool of my basement in Colorado Springs, typing this chapter on my notebook computer, and enjoying the fact that I feel pleasantly satisfied after my LCR breakfast. I also am particularly enjoying the new pants with their 33 inch waist size into which I now comfortably fit!

My weight is stabilized at 179 pounds (plus or minus two pounds depending on whether I am using my "having fun getting on the scale regimen"). I can report that the waist size of my pants has shrunk between 13 and 15 inches (depending on the brand of the pants) in about 12 months. Best of all from an eating comfort standpoint, I have not dieted (gone hungry) but, instead, have feasted.

As detailed in this book, I eat up to eight meals per day: Usually less – it's just too much work to eat all that food!

4. Why The Difference Between Then and Now?

To make the long story short, I simply – as a result of my wife's initial choice to change her grocery shopping selections – changed my eating pattern to the LCR.

Within a few months I noticed dramatic changes in my weight and vitality. I received a kind of "trickle down nutrition" by simply eating the lower carb foods on hand.

Having struggled with weight for years, and having a "why does it work?" kind of mind, I began delving into the research and organizations that support the LCR.

5. The Ultimate Reason for This Book

While serving clients in my practice as a CPA (before I taught Math/NSA/CIS/Business for a local technical college and then ultimately became a fulltime secondary Math Teacher) I worked with two separate groups that were broadly concerned with nutrition and health. Exposure to these groups got me interested in alternative approaches to healthful lifestyles.

I also found that most of us have a need to identify with a cause that we have found works for us and that has the potential to benefit others. One person I met in my life-journey described cause-oriented work as "one beggar telling another where to find food."

So here I am – one "beggar" to another – and I am telling you that the concepts in this book are "food" for health!

VIII. Having fun with weight loss

So much for the background facts. Up to this point we haven't had a lot of fun with our LCR. Let's have some fun now!

- How would you like to never be truly hungry (assuming you can obtain the suggested foods)? Do not panic – for most these foods are not difficult to obtain!

- How would you like to feast on up to eight meals per day?

- How would you like to discover that food flavours now explode with amazing fulfillment in your mouth?

- How would you like to lose weight while you are doing all this eating? (This was a REALLY big plus for me!)

- How would you like to increase your vitality and sense of well-being?

- How would you like to wear significantly "thinner" clothes? (This assumes that you are currently overweight or obese.)

- How would you like to help prevent a pre-diabetic condition that affects or is likely to affect a majority of Americans?

- How would you like to reduce your propensity toward – not only diabetes – but also toward hypertension, certain heart diseases, certain forms of cancer and various other maladies?

These are all possible benefits from a properly followed LCR!

Let's get started!

Chapter Two

Getting Started in Your Low-Carb Eating Regimen

Subsequent chapters in this book will provide a more in-depth view of the actual steps of the Low-Carb Regimen. The current chapter provides a quick overview of the process.

I. The principles behind the Low-Carb Regimen (LCR) are straight-forward:

Changing the way we eat from a conventional high carb, low fat, low protein diet to a correctly followed 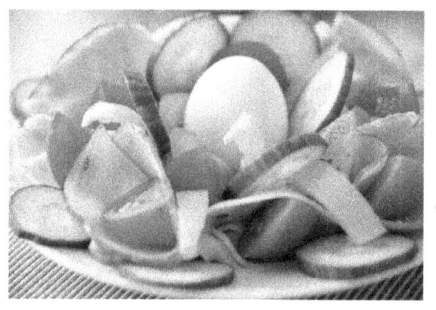 Low-Carb Regimen (LCR) low-carb, high healthful fat, high protein diet can establish a fat-burning metabolism within the average person.

In order to establish this fat-burning metabolism (as opposed to the fat-accumulating metabolisms that plague most people), you will want to:

1. Overcome your addiction to highly refined, high carb foods.

Note: Carbohydrates are foods that readily convert into blood sugar (glucose) in human metabolism.

Carbohydrates are broadly classed as sugars, starches or fiber. Examples of carbohydrate rich foods are grains, pastas, breads, cakes, cookies, pies, sweeteners, starchy vegetables (such as potatoes) and fruits (although, among fruits, berries and melons are relatively low in carbohydrate). Highly refined, high carb foods are the processed carbohydrates such as candies, candy bars, cakes, Ding-Dongs, Ho-Hos, Twinkies, cookies, pies, muffins, pancakes, breads, pastas and cinnamon rolls.

2. Convert your body to a fat-burning metabolism

. . . by eating low-carb, high protein, high healthful fat foods.

Note: Proteins tend to be meats, poultry and eggs (though there are vegetable and dairy proteins). Fats are in foods like bacon (also a protein), real butter and cream rich dairy products (Be careful here: Milk is high carb and ice-cream is high carb as a result of added sugar and milk content).

3. Fuel your fat-burning metabolism

. . . by consistently eating protein and healthful fats while minimizing carbs.

4. Support your fat-burning metabolism

. . . with moderate aerobic exercise and by eliminating strenuous exercise (This is VERY important since strenuous exercise can "shut down" a fat-burning metabolism).

5. Track your progress.

6. Refine your regimen

. . . with appropriate variety and by adding back certain higher-carb foods (as you reach Step Four of the Low-Carb Regimen) that prove to be beneficial to your specific nutritional needs.

7. Learn to maintain your regimen for a lifetime.

II. Here is a quick overview of what I do:

1. I am eating high protein and high healthful fat foods:

For instance, I eat all the steak, chicken, pork, lamb, seafood, protein-in-general (including eggs and bacon!!!), leafy green vegetables, broccoli, asparagus, stir fry, Bell peppers, dry-roasted almonds, butter!!!, sour cream, cream cheese, other cheeses, low-carb yogurt (check out **King Soopers "Carb Control" brand yogurt** – wow, the flavours and the low cost!), **Mission Carb Balance small fajita style tortillas**, strawberries and blueberries (in moderate amounts) that I desire.

I avoid carbohydrates like the plague (unless they are offset by a like count in fiber within the original food itself). I'm learning to bake – I like to cook – with almond flour, coconut flour, milled flax seed, and with chia seeds. Pumpkin pie filling (watch out for the condensed milk!) can be great – just find a low-carb crust (or skip the crust altogether – see the **1 To 5 Low-Carb Cooking Guide** at the end of this book)!

2. This means I minimize the following high carb foods:

All potatoes, corn, breads, buns (including hamburger and hotdog buns), rolls, croissants, crackers, chips, cookies, pie crusts, pizza crusts, Twinkies, Ding Dongs, Ho-Hos, pastas, popcorns, sugars and fruits (strawberries and blueberries are ok – they are reasonably low-carb!) are carbohydrates – I am seeking to cutback on these wherever possible.

Good News: Per the link above, Mission makes commonly available Carb-Balance small fajita style tortillas from which you can make sandwiches, roll ups, fajitas, quesadillas, etc.! We like the "small-fajita" eight count package of Carb Balance whole wheat tortillas: Each tortilla has 13 grams of carbs less 10 grams of fiber for a net carb count of only 3 grams!

As noted, I'm seeking to minimize carbs and in the process I'm finding some real surprises.

For instance, I am astonished at how many grams of carbohydrates are in milk and even in some high fiber foods like chili beans: We are not eating as much chili as we did before and when we make it now we use half as many beans and serve smaller portions of the chili.

Don't get the idea, however, that we are losing out: We are feasting on all the other "non-carb rich" foods that we want along with the more modest portions of chili!

Stuffed to the gills is the way we tend to feel after feasting, though – to be honest – it is more fun and much more beneficial to eat appropriately (until you are full) than it is to overeat.

Keep in mind, you don't need as much at each meal when you regularly eat more frequently!

III. A change in thinking helped me make the change:

In order to embrace change, we need something that has appeal.

Along these lines, years ago a friend taught me that when it comes to effective marketing, we sell the sizzle not the steak!

Try an experiment: Would you rather have a portion of USDA grade A Choice beef, or would you like to have a fresh-off-the-grill, sizzling, mouth watering, succulent, seasoned-to-perfection Porterhouse garnished with all the fixings? No contest, right?

When it comes to eating, our taste buds are consumers that need some marketing. Our taste imaginations need

to be titillated and stimulated to nutritional ecstasy –
then we won't be hungry because we truly will be
satisfied!

1. Seeing false foods for what they are:

Let me offer a caveat: You can't substitute that which is
NOT food for that which is. So much of what our brains
have been trained to regard as good and tasty has the
nutritional value of chalk.

Consider the carb-rich culture and marketing that
inundate our society. These are empty foods that
promote obesity because they stimulate fat production
AND they bar from their rightful place the healthful,
nutritious foods that our bodies desperately need. Once
these food impostors sit in the urge-to-eat driving seats
of our appetites, then we lose sight of the nutritional
destination that dining is really all about.

Mick Jager of the Rolling Stones sang, "I can't get no,
satisfaction . . . "

The context of the song was not nutrition, but the
expression certainly rings true with the American diet.

2. Real nutritional satisfaction:

Let me give you another example: Last night I got
inspired and prepared **a feast** for my spouse. The meal
took me about half an hour to prepare. It was low cost
and so unbelievably tasty, flavourful, aromatically
delicious, and appealing to the eye that my spouse and

I are still savouring it today! Low-Carb Regimen leftovers for lunch, mmmm!

For ideas on your own low-carb feasts, see the **1 To 5 Low-Carb Cooking Guide** in the back of this book.

IV. How to manage your eating:

> **1. There is a huge idea here – Eat until you are full, not until you are stuffed (you will eat again in a few hours!):**

People who diet tend to look at each meal as being like travelling when you come to the last gas station before a five hundred mile stretch in the desert. Under these circumstances, you definitely want to tank up!

> **2. In the Low-Carb Regimen you will NOT be hungry since you dine every few hours.**

So don't expand your stomach by eating each meal as if it were your last – under the Low-Carb Regimen you may eat up to eight meals in a day.

> **3. Therefore, go easy on the portions and eat until you are full – not until you are stuffed!**

So, in all of this we are trying to cut back on carbs, but how do we keep track of the carbs?

V. How to count carbs:

1. There are three critical things that must be known in order to properly count carbs.

First, what quantity of the item in the package constitutes "a portion?"

If the package has twelve ounces, and if two ounces are a portion, then there are six portions in that package. Therefore, if you consume the entire package, you consume six portions worth!

Second, how many grams of carbohydrates are there per portion?

Third, how many grams of fiber are there per portion?

2. Now, subtract the grams of fiber from the grams of carbohydrates (allowing for the number of portions you will consume): These are your net carbs!

3. Our carb target:

The Low-Carb Regimen proposes a beginning target of sixty to eighty grams of carbs per day for those getting started in the new regimen. An ongoing target of fifty grams of carbs per day is desirable and sustainable.

4. Keep the crunch; lose the carbs:

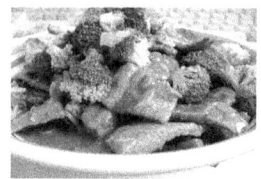The great thing about stir-fry is all that crunching. Great salads have lots of crunch (go light on the carrots, though – they are high carb if eaten in quantity). Red, green, yellow and orange Bell peppers are awesome in salads, great as finger foods, wonderful in stir fry, and I especially love to sauté Bell pepper strips along with sweet onions. Wow, what a side dish, and so good with fresh chicken feta and spinach sausage from Sprouts Market!

Back to the point, here: There is something psychologically satisfying about the message crunchy foods send to the nutrition centers of the brain. Keep in mind that in our new food regimen, food can take longer to eat because of all the crunching (and check out the research on the benefits of chewing – rather than – gulping food)!

5. Sugars and substitute sugars:

Some argue that all sweeteners – artificial and natural – behave in the body like carbohydrates. In the initial months of my Low-Carb Regimen (LCR) when I used sweetener, I used the granulated form of Splenda. I have since switched to both the granulated and liquid forms of **Stevia** (arguably a more natural sugar substitute) depending on the food application to which the sweetener is applied.

6. Milk:

I found a decent replacement for milk in my latte (milk is loaded with carbs and is a problem for the lactose intolerant). Almond and coconut milk (my spouse is allergic to soy) are decent alternatives for many things, but the almond milk and the sweetened version of the coconut milk have an odd taste when I make my latte!

On the other hand I found that the **unsweetened, unflavoured coconut milk** (two grams of carbs less one gram of fiber for a net carb count of only one for an eight ounce glass) makes an acceptable latte. Evidently – over the long-run – as I consumed less carbs, my taste buds adjusted themselves so that I now enjoy low-carb flavours more than ever!

7. Read the label carefully:

In looking for baking alternatives for things like pancakes, I got all excited when I found "Atkins All Purpose Bake Mix" until I read the ingredients: wheat gluten and soy. My spouse is allergic to soy and appears to be allergic to gluten, so this product will not work for us.

On the other hand, if you are not allergic to soy and gluten, this product may be alright for you. However, each one third cup serving is eleven grams of carbs with six grams of fiber (for a net carb count of five grams per one third cup serving). In addition, each serving contains twenty grams of protein – but, still, the carb count is too high for me when each portion is only two and two thirds ounces.

There is a very high fiber flour named **CarbQuik** that is marketed by Netrition. One cup of this flour contains only 6 net grams of carbs. It makes great pancakes and can be used in recipes where flour is required. However, it turns into a "semi-liquid oatmeal consistency" when fluids are added. Accordingly, it is not useful for breads or crusts that you would traditionally knead or roll out. Nonetheless, this flour is a tremendous boost to low-carb cooking efforts!

A caution regarding CarbQuik: This flour may create "carb-craving" (something we work diligently to overcome in Step One of our Low-Carb Regimen). As a result, use of this flour may be better applied in Step Four where we seek to add back certain higher-carb foods that are also low-glycemic.

8. Coffee:

Some within the low-carb movement chide those of us who are still hooked on lattes: The argument tends to be that appropriate nutrition more than replaces the energy craving that is temporarily satisfied by coffee. I'm still working on this: I've always joked that I was born with a caffeine deficiency! More to the point at hand, a plain cup of coffee is zero carbs. For those who require cream a relatively low-carb option is a tablespoon of non-whipped, heavy whipping cream or (even lower-carb, though not as thick) some unsweetened-unflavoured coconut milk. If a sweetener is required, we will – of course – use liquid or granulated Stevia. For a broader discussion on coffee and other beverages, see Chapter Twelve in this book for **Things To Drink Right Now**.

Along with this, have you noticed all the advertised "research" – sponsored by Starbucks, I suspect – touting the benefits of drinking coffee? To me, this is just one more example of the cyclic, marketing driven reports of nutritional "trends" in America.

http://www.webmd.com/food-recipes/features/coffee-new-health-food

VI. The Atkins Diet and the Low-Carb Regimen (LCR):

Dr. Atkins promoted a low-carb diet as an effective weight-loss tool. The popularity of his approach has been built by his successors into a highly structured "movement" with "approved" practitioners and a relatively rigid set of procedures.

The Low-Carb Regimen (LCR) – the subject of this book – is a lifestyle approach whose aim is effective, ongoing weight-loss that supports the elimination of insulin resistance for the "average" participant who does not need medical intervention in order to change their diet.

It seems reasonable that for most, eating a proper diet – in spite of the perils of our carbaholic society – should not require a prescription from a medical professional!

1. Calorie counting may be ineffective in the long run:

There are those who speak against calorie counting and argue that it has not been demonstrated to be effective. Supporting this argument is the fact that even the most highly advertised calorie counting plans appear to have only limited success over the long run (periods greater than two years) when the goal is losing and keeping off the weight.

a) What is a Calorie?

According to Livestrong.com:

"The calorie was originally defined as a unit of heat in 1824 and was later redefined to be a unit of energy. The food calorie represents 1,000 times more energy than the (non-food) calorie and is also known as the kilocalorie. The joule was adopted as the preferred unit of energy for scientific applications in 1948 by the Ninth General Conference on Weights and Measures and formally approved in 1960 by the International System of Units."

The Livestrong.com article goes on to explain:

"The food calorie doesn't represent a precise quantity of energy because its measurement will always include experimental error. In addition, the specific procedure used for determining the energy in a food calorie isn't well standardized since it's no longer a scientific unit of measure. The experimentally observed values for the food calorie range from 4,182 joules to 4,204 joules, depending primarily on the initial conditions used in the test."

Here is the reference where you can read more:

http://www.livestrong.com/article/40175-calorie/#ixzz2VJMsoGHY

Just from the definition of "food calorie," the rationale for counting carbs becomes apparent:

- Calories are not a precise measurement

- Our bodies are NOT Bunsen burners

(we do NOT convert food to energy in the same way measured by researchers)

- Carbs, not calories, may be the "triggers" for body fat accumulation

(our bodies readily convert carbohydrates to glucose which – if we have developed resistance to the insulin that transports the glucose – then ultimately can end up stored as fat).

Carbohydrates, then (and not "food calories") may be the key factors for overweight and obese conditions in the insulin resistant.

In addition, since many – but certainly not all – food calories are contained in highly refined, high carb foods, reducing calories can potentially reduce carb count. Even so, counting calories is unlikely to produce the low-carb regimen necessary for activating a fat-burning metabolism. To emphasize this point again, a properly followed low-carb regimen is needed to establish the fat-burning metabolism that – in turn – allows weight-loss without dieting.

Accordingly, when we participate in the Low-Carb Regimen (LCR), we count carbs – not calories.

2. Fat (in foods – NOT on me!) is my friend:

To begin with, the flavour of foods is in their fat. This is why fat-free foods tend to have the appeal of stale cardboard. When I eat foods containing healthful fat (along with low-carb and high protein foods), my metabolism doesn't have to accumulate excess body fat!

On the other hand, if you want to be fat (and if you are insulin resistant), eat highly refined, high carb foods!

Conversely, if you want to return to your appropriate weight (and if you are insulin resistant), lay off the carbs and follow the Low-Carb Regimen (LCR) . . . and do NOT starve yourself. Eat at reasonable times (every two to four hours) when you are hungry.

3. How often we eat:

In the Low-Carb Regimen we feast up to eight meals per day.

It is actually a bit of work to eat this often, but it is worth the effort.

There are occasions when a more elaborate low-carb meal is not practical. In these instances a "meal" might be just a pack of **Emerald Dry Roasted Almonds**, and/or a few strips of bacon supplemented with some cheese.

"Wait a minute," you say (again!) – "this is only a snack."

In response I note that whether you call it a snack, or not, in the Low-Carb Regimen (LCR) it is a meal.

Along these lines, there is an old Abraham Lincoln story: Mr. Lincoln inquired of some friends, "What if I told you that a horse's tail is a leg and then asked you how many legs the horse has?" Mr. Lincoln reported that his friends responded, "Well, we suppose then, five legs." To which Mr. Lincoln observed, "No, only four legs – it doesn't matter what you call it, a horse's tail is still only a tail."

4. Exercise for the right purpose and at the right time:

Conventional wisdom says that – if we want to reduce our waistline – we need to cut back on calories AND exercise regularly (many interpret "regularly" as "strenuously"). For the insulin resistant, however, these approaches may be counter-productive. What we want is to healthfully get out bodies to stop storing fat (frequently a major problem for the insulin resistant). When we cut back on calories, our bodies can enter into a "starvation mode" which actually may stimulate fat retention. Strenuous exercise – as opposed to light aerobic exercise – may produce a similar result.

In other words, people want to lose weight so they eat less and exercise more strenuously, and (for the insulin resistant) they could end up merely gaining – or at least not losing – weight. On the other hand following this book's "feasting" regimen (I do NOT diet!), may decrease the propensity of the body to retain fat and may stimulate weight-loss and energy increase (along with a host of other potential health benefits).

VII. Understanding the Low-Carb Regimen (LCR) "Jargon"

Every significant human endeavour tends to develop its own vocabulary or "jargon."

Those who enjoy baking, football, painting, volleyball, car racing, mountain biking, etc., all use vocabulary unique to their specific pursuit. As you might expect, it is no less so in the world of low-carb eating.

Here are some terms that will help your understanding of the concepts in this book:

- Atkins diet - The most widely known low-carb diet was originated by Dr. Robert Atkins who based his ideas upon the work of Kekwick and Pawain and Dr. Alfred Pennington. This diet has become highly commercialized and is noted for its extreme "Induction Phase" in which carbs are reduced to 20 grams per day. This diet also fails to focus on insulin resistance as a major contributor to obesity in America.

- Body Mass Index – A numeric index designed to identify "underweight, normal, overweight and obese ranges."

- BMI – Acronym (initials) for "Body Mass Index."

- carb (short for "carbohydrate") – An abbreviation of "grams of carbohydrate."

- carb count – A measure of the number of grams of carbohydrate in a specific food.

- fat – Dietary fats are one of three major categories of food (along with proteins and carbohydrates). The generally accepted nutritional view is that saturated fats and trans fats are associated with raising your cholesterol levels and increasing your risk for heart disease. On the other hand, monounsaturated fats and polyunsaturated fats are thought to lower cholesterol and reduce your risk of heart disease. In general, fats consist of a wide group of compounds that will dissolve in organic solvents but not in water. Fats in the body may be seen as triglycerides: tri-esters of glycerol and any of several fatty acids. Fat is technically a subset of a group known as lipids. "Oils" is usually used to refer to fats that are liquids at normal room temperature, while "fats" is usually used to refer to fats that are solids at normal room temperature. "Lipids" is used to refer to both liquid and solid fats, along with other related substances, usually in a medical or biochemical context.

- fat-burning metabolism – The popular description for keto-lipolysis. Keto-lipolysis is the term used to describe a metabolism that "fuels itself" by converting fat stores into energy.

- fiber – One of three subcategories of carbohydrate along with sugars and starches. Fibers are not normally absorbed nutritionally.

- glucose – The blood sugar result of metabolized (processed within our bodies) carbohydrate (foods containing sugar, starches and/or fiber). Examples of carbohydrate include grains, breads, sweets, pastries, pastas, fruits potatoes and other starchy vegetables.

- glycemic index – A number indicating the expected blood sugar (glucose) impact of a food. The scale rates glucose at 100. The closer foods are to 100, the higher their glycemic impact.

- high glycemic – A more technical way of saying that the food has a high sugar (glucose) impact in our bodies.

- ideal body weight – Generally about a ten pound range on the Body Mass Index (BMI) scale in which we are neither underweight, overweight nor obese.

- insulin – A hormone created by the pancreas beta cells that is released into the blood stream in order to transport glucose to our cells for energy.

- insulin resistance – A condition ("conditions" set the stage for disease) in which the cells in our body "reject" excess glucose and store it as fat (especially around the belly). Insulin resistance is considered a pre-diabetic condition and is associated with major disease including Type II diabetes, heart disease, hypertension and certain forms of cancer. Insulin resistance tends to respond well to a low-carb diet.

- keto-genesis – A descriptor for the creation of a fat-burning metabolism.

- keto-lipolysis – A descriptor for a fat-burning metabolism.

- ketosis – The term most commonly used among low-carb dieters to describe a fat-burning metabolism. **Ketosis** actually means an elevated state of ketone bodies in the body as a whole. This is frequently associated with elevated ketone levels in the bloodstream (a by-product of a fat-burning metabolism).

- Low-Carb Regimen (LCR) – The dietary regimen described in this book.

- net carbs – Total grams of carbohydrates less the grams of fiber actually contained in the original carbohydrate (adding additional grams of pure fiber only adds a like amount of carbohydrate for a zero change in net carbs).

- overweight – As a rule of thumb, the first twenty pounds in excess of the upper limit for an ideal weight per the Body Mass Index (BMI) scale. Generally, the upper limit for an ideal weight on the BMI scale is 25.

- obese – In common usage the word means "considerably overweight." More formally, the word "obese" is used to describe specific ranges above 25 on the Body Mass Index (BMI) scale.

- protein – In our common experience proteins are meats, poultry, eggs and seafood. However, there are proteins in vegetables and dairy products, as well.

- starch – The non-sugar, non-fiber component of carbohydrate.

- sugar – The subdivision of carbohydrate that is most readily converted to glucose within human metabolism.

Chapter Two Conclusion:

Chapters One and Two are now complete! In them we have a sufficient foundation in our weight-loss without dieting to launch with understanding into the first of The Five Steps of the Low-Carb Regimen (LCR)!

Chapter Three

Step One of Five:

Overcoming Carb Withdrawal

In this chapter we introduce the steps (phases) of the Low-Carb Regimen (LCR) that allow us to move from weight-loss without dieting to ongoing maintenance of a healthy weight throughout our lives. Key to this process is establishing a "fat-burning" metabolism. However, those who seek to establish a "fat-burning" metabolism must first overcome their addiction to highly refined, high carb foods. The addictive nature of highly refined, high carb foods causes a mild withdrawal for most who eliminate such foods. This is why it is necessary to overcome carb withdrawal.

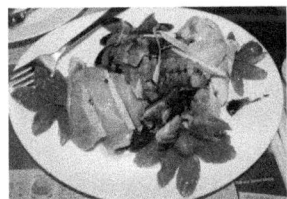

Step One – Overcoming Carb Withdrawal presents the "step-by-stop" process required to succeed in defeating addiction to high glycemic carbs.

I. An Oveview Of The Low-Carb Regimen (LCR)

1. The Five Steps Are:

a) Step One – Overcoming carb withdrawal

b) Step Two – Activating a fat burning metabolism

c) Step Three – Optimizing our low-carb regimen

d) Step Four – Including select previously excluded foods

e) Step Five – Maintaining a Low-Carb Eating Regimen for a lifetime

As noted before, overcoming carb withdrawal requires dramatic eating regimen changes for the typical American carbaholic diet. However, while extreme low-carb eating is useful in "kick starting" a fat-burning metabolism, over the long run it may deprive our bodies of essential nutrients. This is where pacing (a process built into the five steps) comes in.

2. At The Right Time We Will Re-introduce Beneficial Higher Carb Foods:

Ultimately – although eliminating high glycemic (highly refined high carb) foods is something to do for a lifetime – eliminating essential nutrients is not.

In a lifetime of healthy eating and appropriate weight maintenance it is not advisable to avoid ALL foods that may have higher carbohydrate counts.

As an example, apples – though high carb – have some wonderful nutrients AND we can eat just half an apple in a day instead of one or more apples. In the same way, modest portions of whole grains, beans and other legumes can be incorporated into our diets as we reach our weight loss goals. The key in this is timing: We avoid and minimize certain high carb foods as we establish a fat-burning metabolism and we re-introduce those healthful, moderately higher carb foods in moderate portions as we seek to maintain our weight loss advances.

II. Required Background For Step One: Overcoming Carb Withdrawal

1. Correcting Our Thinking about Overcoming Carb Withdrawal:

Most of us begin the LCR as hardcore carbohydrate addicts.

Sadly, most of us also do not realize to what extent we are addicted to high carb and highly refined high carb foods.

Sugar-laden cheesecakes, ice creams, cookies, candies, chocolate confections, black forest cakes, cakes in general along with their icings, sugary beverages, sodas, pies, bagels, pretzels, pizzas and foods that are "starchy or sweet in general" tend to rule the lives of most in America. Is it any wonder that obesity is rampant?

When the truth is told it becomes apparent that most of us are so addicted that we feel we absolutely have to have our pasta, potatoes, breads, corn and other starchy vegetables (these are all high carb foods). Without being aware of the carb overload, we become addicted to high carb fruit juices, high carb fruits, chocolate beverages (almost all are loaded with high glycemic sugars) and other high carb "beverages."

Further, we tend to be shocked to discover that the high carb verdict includes most smoothies and most "meal replacement" and protein shakes.

When we look at "buying into" a low-carb eating regimen, the high carb "sticker shock" may appear to some as an unimaginably high cost – a cost made even worse when we discover that even common, dairy based milks in all their variations of milk fat are high carb.

There goes the latte! (Hold your judgment on this: Good news is coming!)

"What's left?" we might think. Are we to survive on gruel and the distantly dreamed of aroma of those high carb and highly refined high carb foods mentioned above?

This tends to be the initial mindset of many who seek to begin a Low-Carb Regimen.

2. Good News in the Overcoming Carb Withdrawal Step:

- **Good News:** As we begin our LCR – for many – physical carb withdrawal tends to last only two to four days.

Note: It is possible that our bodies may react to carb withdrawal with responses – normally mild – associated with reversing addictions. Obviously, if we experience significant health concerns, we will address these to those medically trained to deal with them. Typically, however, the worst one experiences in carb withdrawal is a short-lived desire for the high carb foods that we are replacing with healthful and delicious low-carb, high fat, high protein alternatives.

- **Good news:** We do NOT go hungry – ever!

Note: It is common, however, to occasionally yearn for some high carb loaded food: Use your **Will Power and Planning** for Successful Weight Loss strategies – discussed a bit further into this current chapter – to replace carb yearning with yearning for healthful low-carb alternatives.

- **Good news: We do NOT diet – we feast on absolutely delicious foods.**

- **Good news: We feast up to eight times per day.**

With all this good news, then, how do we begin to overcome carb withdrawal?

3. Lifestyle Changes in the Overcoming Carb Withdrawal Step:

For many, the overcoming carb withdrawal step – the first step – is the hardest to take.

- This is the step that requires a paradigm shift (a major re-alignment) in our thinking.

- This is the step that requires lifestyle changes that support – and do not thwart – establishing a fat burning metabolism.

- This is the step that requires planning for success by rearranging our food purchasing, our food preparation and our food ingestion (dining) process.

- This is the step that requires planning to insure that we do not allow ourselves to go hungry.

- This is the step that requires dealing with the cravings that can come from carb withdrawal.

In short, these steps are the lifestyle changes that actually can shift our metabolism from a fat storage process (CGI: carbohydrate-glucose-insulin) to a fat-burning (keto-lipolysis, or – more commonly – ketosis) energy cycle. For more on this, see the section in Chapter Four on **How to Know** If You Have Developed a Fat Burning Metabolism.

4. Will Power and Planning for Successful Weight Loss:

According to a **recent article**, individuals perceived to have will power exercise that will power by planning and putting into place mechanisms for success. In the case of low-carb weight loss, those with will power will insure that low-carb alternatives are in place (including in place at work!) and ready to eat before beginning their lifestyle change.

This also means that these foods – for instance, bell pepper strips, slices of cheese, deviled eggs, packets of **dry roasted almonds, Krogers Carbmaster yogurt** containers, microwaveable (pre-cooked) bacon and previously prepared meat (beef strips, chicken, etc.) – are in your house and ready to go when you are. I even keep packets of dry roasted almonds in my car, by my bed and beside my favourite "watching TV" chair!

Keep in mind that one of the best ways to keep from eating highly refined high carb foods (breads, cakes, pies, pastries, etc.) is to plan to stay out of the bakery

5. Re-invigorating Our Taste Buds:

An extraordinary change that takes place in the LCR is the discovery of how wonderfully good food can actually taste. I believe part of the reason that the flavour of food seems to explode in our mouths as never before – once we've adopted the Low-Carb Regimen – is a "re-invigoration" of our taste buds. This makes sense when we consider that the constant

barrage of highly refined high carbohydrate foods in the modern diet appears to dull the ability of our "flavour processing" capacity to respond to food.

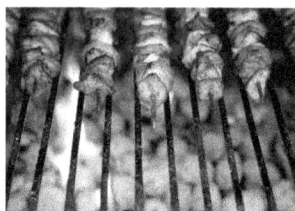 Along these lines, it is a common occurrence for those adopting a low-carb diet to speak with surprised delight about how delicious their meals now taste. This is not really surprising, though, when one considers how "exhausted and overcome" our taste bud receptors must become when continually bombarded with highly refined high carb foods!

It is important to note, then, that the phenomenon of food now tasting much better does not result from appreciating food more "because you get so little of it" (a complete misconception regarding the Low-Carb Regimen!). Keep in mind that we do NOT go hungry in the LCR. Instead, we feast!

6. This Is NOT Atkins:

In the Atkins approach, the overcoming process is referred to as **Induction**.

There are key and critical differences between the LCR and Atkins.

For instance, the LCR has at its core the goal of removing the "fuel" (highly refined, high carb "foods") for insulin resistance. (Insulin resistance is described in greater detail in **Chapter Fifteen**.)

In addition, the Atkins goal is to "shock" the system by an abrupt eating regimen shift from a typical highly refined high carb diet that may be several hundred grams or more of net carbs each day to an extreme low-carb diet (20 grams of net carbs per day). I believe, however, that for many – if not for most – this is unnecessarily abrupt.

Instead, I believe that it is both possible and desirable to adopt a LCR more gradually. See the recent JAMA articles on low-carb dieting for more information regarding this.

Another unique feature of the LCR is that it initially seeks to limit net carb counts to a range of 60 to 80 grams of carbs daily. Then – once this is achieved – the goal becomes 50 grams of net carbs daily.

III. How We Achieved The Overcoming Carb Withdrawal Step, Week-By-Week

As a foundational concept we learned to NOT let ourselves get hungry. We did this by eating smaller, more frequent meals (up to eight times per day!). We discovered that dry roasted almonds are delicious and very filling. See the section of this book dealing with **Things to Eat Right Now**.

1. Week One:

We began by cutting back on potatoes, pastas, cereals and breads. This process was not difficult because we

were able to substitute other more healthful, more nutritious, more delicious, lower carb foods! To see the foods that we began to eat, check out the sections of this book covering: **Things to Eat Right Now**, **Things to Drink Right Now**, and **Where's the Bread**?.

This did require some serious adjustments in our eating regimen. I remember complaining to my students (I teach high school students Mathematics) that "I get no potatoes" (though I was not the least bit hungry).

During this first week we also replaced sugar with Stevia and sought to reduce the use of sweeteners wherever we could. For the most part, we eliminated sodas.

2. Week Two:

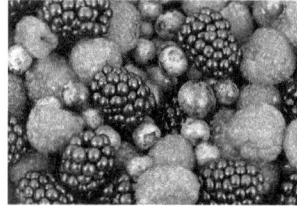 In week two, high carb fruits, juices and protein/meal replacement shakes and smoothies had to go. This was made so much easier because we replaced the high carb fruits with modest portions of strawberries, blueberries, raspberries and melons.

3. Week Three:

In week three I was able to replace dairy milk. It was – for me – a huge step when I replaced milk in my lattes (normally two each day) with unsweetened, unflavoured coconut milk. As noted before, since a cup of milk contains 12 net grams of carbs (while a cup of

unsweetened, unflavoured coconut milk is only 1 net gram of carbs), this allowed me to save 22 net grams of carbs per day. Wow!

- We also reviewed our diet for "hidden" carbs.

- We learned to select low-carb options when we dined out in local restaurants: You don't have to eat the bread and the potatoes that restaurants serve AND you can select a chicken Caesar salad for your entree (ask for oil and vinegar dressing)!

- We learned to shop for the right low-carb foods and to make certain that highly refined high carb options had no place in our pantry.

- We made certain that high carb vegetables were eliminated from our eating regimen.

- We checked our cooking supplies to ensure that the healthful low-carb foods required to eat LCR delicious were on hand and in good stock.

- We began expanding our recipes to include the mouth watering low-carb, high fat, high protein foods described in this book and in the **1 To 5 Low-Carb Cooking Guide**.

By this time our fat burning metabolisms (keto-lipolysis) were producing the desired results of weight loss, energy increase and a much greater sense of well-being. We were excited at how easy, how enjoyable and how productive the entire process actually was, and we began planning for new, smaller sized clothes to fit body frames that became increasingly more fit.

4. For The Weeks Thereafter:

We ate and continue to feast on the most flavourful and satisfying meals I can ever recall eating. I love my breakfast of two eggs over easy with two strips of bacon. For variety, I make omelettes or scrambled eggs.

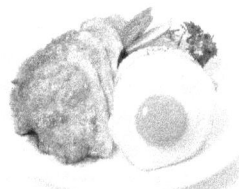 Not enough, you say? I also get my large latte, berries or melons if I wish them and – if I wish to indulge – a slice of one of my wonderful homemade, low-carb breads loaded with butter. If I'm still hungry by the time I have my second latte, I finish off with some dry roasted almonds. When I eat all this, I'm so full I'm ready to waddle!

5. For Your Lifetime:

Something amazing begins to happen here: As our saggy, stretched out stomachs slowly and painlessly (we don't allow ourselves to get truly hungry in this Low-Carb Regimen) shrink, we need less food to feel full. Although we can eat as much as we want (of healthful low-carb, high healthful fat, high protein foods), we simply want less. We must not, however, allow ourselves to go hungry or to go without food every few hours.

In summary then, the description above is how we have achieved the benefits of a low-carb, high fat, high protein lifestyle.

As anyone who has succeeded in this effort tends to feel: If we did it, so can you!

Let's now look at how to know when we have succeeded in Step One - Overcoming Carb Withdrawal. In addition, let's look at the mental and emotional aspects of carb craving with some very practical means of dealing with these problems (including eating Italian!).

IV. How to Know When You Have Succeeded in Overcoming Physical Carb Withdrawal

Before we launch into a discussion of the remaining four steps, let's address how to know when we have completed the "Overcoming" step.

It is important to keep in mind that our goal in the Overcoming Step is to eliminate our physical addiction to high carb and highly refined high carb foods. When our bodies no longer physically crave these high glycemic carbohydrates (foods that spike our blood sugar levels) – evidenced by our ongoing lifestyle shift

---

to a low-carb eating regimen – then we have the needed demonstration of success in our Step One: Overcoming process.

This step eliminates the physical, but not necessarily the mental and emotional addictions to a carbaholic lifestyle.

1. Overcoming Our Emotional Addiction to Carbohydrates

Over the years most of us have developed emotional coping mechanisms linked to high carbohydrate and highly refined high carb foods. Just think of the images that are seen in the movies. Stereotypically, if a woman is depressed – perhaps as a result of a failed relationship – she is portrayed downing copious quantities of high carb Rocky Road ice cream. Men struggling with discouragement are frequently shown drinking large quantities of high carb alcoholic beverages.

These scenes are common in the American lifestyle. Those adopting a low-carb regimen obviously seek to avoid these kinds of "coping mechanisms."

Consequently – if our coping mechanisms are tied to food and beverage – it is beneficial to have ready those wonderful low-carb eating regimen "special treats" and beverages that allow a low glycemic support for our mental and emotional needs. Uplifting interactions with supportive friends, mild exercise, or helpfully engaging distractions such as a great book, sporting event or multimedia experience are other "low-carb" options.

2. Eating Italian

On the other hand, sometimes we just want Italian. The pasta is the problem. There are no true pastas that are actually low-carb. In addition, low glycemic claims by some pasta manufacturers should be investigated with a wary eye. If the pasta is primarily made with grains (a

requirement for true pasta), then the carb count is high. As explained in the section of this book on **Grasping Net Carb Counts**, the addition of fiber to already high carb count grains does NOT reduce the net carb count. On the other hand, if someone develops a pasta whose primary ingredient is psyllium or milled flax seed, then we might actually enjoy a low-carb plate of spaghetti.

There are options, of course, for those of us who love Italian cuisine.

We can use low-carb – read the labels carefully (only some are low-carb) – diced tomatoes to create marinara and other Italian sauces. Fats are our friends, so we can use great Italian cheeses, olive oils and butter liberally.

They are also unbelievably tasty on chicken dishes and as a component in my lightly fried spinach and diced tomato side dish.

In addition, recipes abound for low-carb pizzas. The crust tends to be the problem, but there are creative alternatives that enable us to continue to enjoy this delightful food.

3. We Need a Treat Right Now (but we need to plan to have it on hand and ready to go!)

a) Blueberry Flax Muffins – just eat half of one! (even a half is only relatively low-carb)

You can find somewhat low-carb high fiber muffins (**Flax4Life brand Wild Blueberry Flax Muffins**: at 16 net grams of carbs per HALF muffin) from Wholefoods and Sprout's Markets. For emphasis, a word of caution on the muffins: They are 32 net grams of carbs for a WHOLE (as opposed to a half) muffin. Much lower carb levels can be obtained if you are willing to bake your own per guidelines suggested in The 1 To 5 Low-Carb Cooking Guide at the end of this book.

b) Almond Logs

Wholefoods and Sprouts Markets along with other stores also offer relatively low-carb almond logs (**Minnie Beasley's Almond Lace**: at 4 net grams of carbs per cookie) and truly low-carb toasted sesame seaweed snacks that taste very much like kettle corn!

c) Low-Carb Tortillas

Mission Carb Balance Small Whole Wheat Fajita Style Tortillas are low-carb and can be enjoyed warmed and rolled up with or without fillings (you may want to make quesadillas).

d) Truly Low-Carb Almonds (not all are!)

Emerald Dry Roasted Almonds are available in inexpensive individual portion packets and are great any time you need crunch and protein.

e) Dress Up Some Celery!

Celery slices are great with crunchy peanut butter, almond butter, cheeses, and cream cheese.

f) Pleasing Parfaits

Remember that you can also enjoy fresh blueberries, raspberries or sliced strawberries over **CarbMaster Yogurt** with whipped topping sprinkled with bakers cocoa (a parfait!). The parfait is a nice help in dealing with chocolate cravings. In addition, unsweetened, unflavored coconut milk – when warmed – combines well with a teaspoon each of baker's cocoa and granulated Stevia (or, a few drops of liquid Stevia). To this I add a few ounces of unwhipped heavy whipping cream to make great hot chocolate. Once the chocolate is sufficiently dissolved, this beverage can be refrigerated if your desire is chocolate milk.

There is absolutely no need to crave carbs either physically, mentally or emotionally!

4. Overcoming Carb Withdrawal Is a Worthy Achievement

When we can consistently feast in our daily eating regimen in such a manner that our appetite is satisfied on the initially allowed 60 to 80 grams of daily net carbs (See the section of this book: **An Overview of Low-carb Eating**), then we have Overcome Carb Withdrawal. It is at this stage that we no longer yearn uncontrollably for high carb and highly refined high carb foods.

We are now able to gladly choose the better path of the low-carb, high healthful fat, high protein eating regimen. These foods are now unbelievably delicious and satisfying to us. We no longer worry about being hungry because we feast every few hours – up to eight times per day!

5. A Foundation for Ongoing Health

Overcoming Carb-Withdrawal is a significant milestone in the low-carb weight-loss without dieting regimen. It means that we no longer "have to have" the high carb and highly refined high carb foods that can enslave our metabolisms into the bondage of being overweight and ultimately obese. It also means that in addition to overcoming a literal "carbaholic" addiction that we are now equipped to deal meaningfully with a host of potentially developing problems. These can include physical conditions that may set the stage for insulin resistance, pre-diabetes, diabetes, elevated blood pressure, heart disease, certain forms of cancer and the numerous related problems that go along with these ailments.

Those already diagnosed with these ailments will – of course – choose to seek the guidance, counsel, and expert care of the medical practitioners who are trained to deal with such issues.

With these things in mind, let us return to the matter of success in Step One: Overcoming Carb Withdrawal. By succeeding in Step One, we have gone from a relatively "powerless" position regarding controlling our weight-loss efforts to a position of "power" in our lifestyle management. Once we overcome carb withdrawal, successful weight-loss without dieting is within our grasp.

Congratulations!

However, achieving the ability to master our eating regimen does NOT in and of itself guarantee weight loss. Activating a fat burning metabolism – a process known as keto-lipolysis or more commonly as ketosis – is a critical step for achieving this result in the Low-Carb Regimen.

Chapter Three Conclusion:

In this current chapter we explored the first of the five LCR Steps: Overcoming Carb Withdrawal.

Subsequent chapters will deal with the other Four Steps: Activating, Optimizing, Including and Maintaining.

As you continue in your journey through the Five Steps of the LCR, your author wishes you good and healthful low-carb eating!

Chapter Four
Step Two of Five
Activating A Fat-Burning Metabolism

As a reminder, The Five Steps of the Low-Carb Regimen (LCR) are:

a) Step One – Overcoming carb withdrawal

b) Step Two – Activating a fat-burning metabolism

c) Step Three – Optimizing our low-carb regimen

d) Step Four – Including select previously excluded foods

e) Step Five – Maintaining a low-carb eating regimen for a lifetime

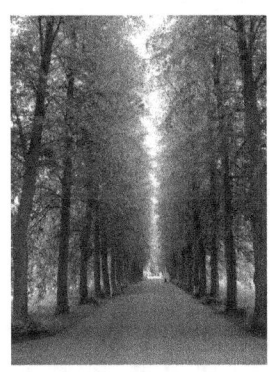

Achieving the ability to master our eating regimen does NOT in and of itself guarantee weight loss.

Activating a fat burning metabolism – a process commonly known as ketosis – is a critical step in our weight-loss without dieting journey.

I. Step Two: Activating a Fat Burning Metabolism

1. Our Objective in Step Two

In our first step we Overcame Carb Withdrawal. With our metabolic foundation "primed" for success, we now focus in earnest on establishing a fat burning metabolism!

2. Refining Our Daily Net Grams of Carbs Intake

While 60 to 80 daily net grams of carbohydrate is the target for our Step One: Overcoming Carb Withdrawal, our Step Two daily target is 50 net grams of carbohydrates. As we reach this goal we should see tangible evidence of keto-lipolysis (a fat burning metabolism) in our systems.

In the Atkins diet the target during the "Induction" phase is a mere 20 net grams of carbohydrate on a daily basis in order to "kick start" ketosis. To generate less stress on our metabolisms, it seems more sensible to look for evidence of a fat-burning metabolism (ketosis) at the higher daily net carb level of 50 grams of net carbs per day. We can always try more severe approaches if moderation fails to produce the results that we seek.

3. Demonstrating That We Have Achieved a Fat Burning Metabolism

We can verify our progress in achieving a fat burning metabolism (ketosis) through the use of **ketone test strips**. In addition, simple biometric readings such as recording our weight and actually measuring our waist can also demonstrate that we are making progress and (in consideration of our low-carb, high fat, high protein eating regimen), therefore, establishing a fat burning metabolism.

In addition, a fat-burning metabolism tends to cause a rather "flowery" smell to urine and a slight "sweetness" in smell to the breath. Though these observations are not as precise as the ketone test strips, they are still indicators of the presence of a fat-burning metabolism.

a) Encapsulating these ideas:

- Those seeking a LCR may want verification that their metabolisms have converted from a glucose energy cycle to a fat burning energy cycle.

- A fat burning metabolism can be a key to weight loss.

- Enabling our metabolisms to shift from a fat creating, excess carbohydrate energy cycle to a (low-carb, high fat, high protein diet) body-fat burning energy cycle is a goal of the LCR.

i) One of the fascinating and measurable by-products of an ongoing fat burning metabolism is the excretion of ketones.

ii) Atkins reported that early researchers (Kekwick and Pawain in the 1950s and 60s) in obesity and fat metabolism identified a "FMS" (fat-mobilizing substance) that appeared in the urine of people whose metabolisms were successfully "burning" body fat.

iii) When this substance was injected into mice, it stimulated the fat "burning" process in the test animals.

c) Which leads to a simple urine test to verify ketone excretion

i) The test involves introducing test strips to urine excretions and then comparing the results against an included colour coded chart.

ii) This is essentially a "litmus" test for ketones.

iii) Here is the link to the "ReliOn Ketone Test Strips" available through Walmart for about seven dollars (50 strips for 50 tests – each test takes about 15 seconds):

walmart.com/ip/Reli-On-Ketone-Test-Strip

iv) Again, the significance is that ketones in the urine are viewed as an indicator that the body's metabolic process is actively burning fat.

4. Having Fun "Stepping on the Scale"

Having a scale in our homes is not as popular as it once was. However, many of us own Wii gaming systems. The Wii Fit Plus program will accurately measure and chart our weight. In addition the software gives an approximate BMI (Body Mass Index) measurement. There are limitations to this program, however. For instance the balance board will not accurately measure weights greater than 330 pounds.

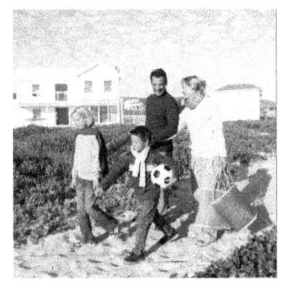 On the positive side – for those of us who find it inconvenient to get out for a walk – the **Wii Fit Plus** program allows simulated walking, jogging and bicycling exercises (along with many other activities) through pleasant virtual worlds. Frankly, it is very nice to be able to roll out of bed and go for a light walk of fifteen to twenty minutes without the need to dress up and without actually leaving the house. Of course, by staying inside you miss the opportunity for Vitamin D benefits, but you don't have to worry about the weather or how "dumpy" you may look that day!

5. Obtaining Useful Weight Measurements

As is commonly experienced, our weight can vacillate with our daily routine. Fluid retention alone can account for a couple of pounds. The old adage is that "a pint (of water) is a pound the world around."

Since it only takes two cups to make a pint, just one glass of water will raise your weight one half of a pound. For this reason, more consistent readings are obtained by taking weight measurements at the same time and in the same circumstances. I put stock in my weekly weight readings, but only casually note my daily readings.

For me, first thing in the morning is useful after excretion/elimination and before food and fluid intake. Keep in mind that on a daily basis it is not unusual to see fluctuations in weight of a fraction of a pound to two or three pounds depending on the accuracy of your scale and other factors. So as noted before, select a day of the week when you can conveniently get a reliable weight measurement and pay attention to your weekly progress.

6. Biometrics: I Like My Belt

The easiest measurement of waist size is our belt. It is a simple matter to note where you notch your belt now and where it is as you make progress toward your weight loss goals. It is also a delight to "have to" go out and purchase smaller sized clothes to fit your trimming body! My closet has the 46 and 48 inch pants I wore at the beginning of my LCR and now contains clothes with a 33 inch waist that I comfortably wear.

Now that's a useful biometric measurement!

7. Be Wary of Low-Carb and Low Glycemic Claims about Processed Foods

A popular player in the low-carb bread market is Julian Bakery's **"Zero Carb" Bread**. A review of its ingredient shows that it is primarily made from psyllium "flour" and organic gluten free oat flour. These small loaves are advertised to have "about" sixteen slices in each loaf, and each slice is reported to have less than one gram of net carbs. My concern is that a mere one third of a cup of oat flour has a net carb count of 16 or more net grams of carbohydrate.

If the "Zero Carb" Bread recipe contains one third of a cup – or more – of the oat flour, then it is unlikely that the "Zero Carb" label is correct.

There are a growing number of reports expressing concern regarding advertised low-carb and/or low glycemic products. Buyers beware!

On the other hand, when you make your own, you can know with confidence the net carb count for your baked items. Baked tend to also be much fresher and – I believe – more tastefully and nutritionally satisfying.

8. Exercise in Low-Carb Weight Loss

As noted before, excessive exercise can work against our weight loss objectives by stimulating our bodies into a "non-ketosis" energy cycle. In addition, muscle is more dense than fat and – as you replace fat with muscle – you increase density and, therefore, weight.

On the other hand, one might argue that they really want the muscle right now. If this is your view, then you must choose between the effective weight loss of the low-carb regimen and the Arnold Swartzenegger muscles. The two goals do not support each other.

For this reason modest exercise –10 to 20 minutes of light aerobic exercise – is encouraged during the weight loss steps (Steps One thru Four) of our low-carb weight loss regimen.

9. Hormonal Balance Shifts

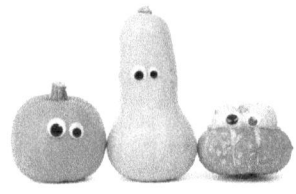

As men lose weight, their hormonal balance tends to shift towards testosterone. This can produce some rather interesting responses to situations. For instance, you really may not want to find the biggest guy around and "clean his clock!" This is hyperbole of course, but the point is be prepared for possible re-orientations of disposition.

This can also lead to increased sex drive which, hopefully, is a good thing.

10. Unfair Advantage for Men

It does tend to be more difficult for women to lose weight and this trend surfaces in the low-carb weight loss without dieting regimen.

The female form is designed for greater protection of the metabolism required for reproduction and child rearing. Thinking back to the prehistory and early history of our species, if there is a famine, stored fat may enable us to survive.

While I enjoyed losing a pound and a half or more of my obese weight each week, a woman in similar circumstances might see only a half pound of weight loss.

Do NOT be discouraged: If we are not gaining weight as we once did, we are at least maintaining and enjoying the enormous benefits of a low-carb regimen.

These include creating a metabolism that can aid in dealing with insulin resistance and the myriad other diseases associated with the overweight/obese lifestyle.

11. If We Are "Stuck"

If you are faithful to the low-carb regimen detailed in this book and yet are not making progress, a visit with a medical practice familiar with low-carb eating regimens is suggested.

Keep in mind that our metabolisms are complex, and "one size does NOT fit all." You may have unique needs that call for the intervention of medical professionals with knowledge of insulin resistance protocols.

II. Net Carbs Counts And Foods That Support A Fat-Burning Metabolism

A. Our bottom line is the net carb count of the foods we eat:

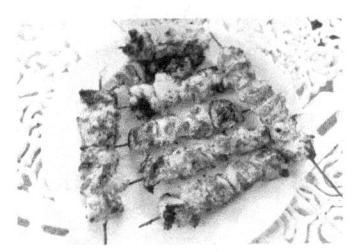 If the net carb count (grams of total carbs less grams of carbs from fiber) is low (a few grams), we can eat it DEPENDING ON the quantity of the food we plan

to eat AND the amount of the food that comprises a portion (read the label!).

Eating high carb foods contributes to a body-fat accumulating energy cycle in our bodies.

B. Our net carb goal:

To overcome carb withdrawal, our daily net carb target was 60 to 80 grams of net carbs per day (See **Chapter Three**: Overcoming Carb Withdrawal).

To establish a fat-burning metabolism our daily carb target is 50 grams of net carbs per day.

This target can be lowered for a few days as needed. However, keep in mind the essential requirement to obtain adequate nourishment each day! The LCR is NOT about starvation: It is, instead, about abundant nutrition through a properly followed eating regimen whose emphasis is low-carb, high healthful fat and high protein foods.

In general, however, if a food is low in carbs, nutritious and you are ready for nourishment – eat it!

Please Note: Traditional dieting is based on limiting food intake (which can lead to the discomfort of hunger). From this perspective the Low-Carb Regimen excludes "dieting" in pursuit of our goal of eating before we become truly hungry. As noted before, in the Low-Carb Regimen we eat up to eight times per day by simply replacing destructive foods with other delicious and more healthful low-carb foods.

C. The following foods are eaten (up to eight times per day!) – this is not an exhaustive list, but it's a good start:

1. Eggs

2. Bacon!

3. Other meats – steak, hamburger, chicken, pork, turkey, lamb, ham, salmon,

other fish, seafood, etc.

4. Nuts (especially almonds)

5. Unsweetened almond and/or unsweetened coconut milk

6. Coffee including lattes made with unflavoured (I find lattes are much better when the coconut milk is unflavoured!), unsweetened coconut milk (I also find lattes are much better with coconut milk than with almond milk). Avoid latte "syrups"

and syrups in general – they are loaded with carbs!

7. Teas including herbal teas

8. Fruit infused waters (but not fruit or vegetable juices). See **Chapter Twelve** to

learn about infused waters and juices.

9. Berries including strawberries, blueberries and raspberries

10. Leafy green vegetables

11. Broccoli, asparagus, cucumbers, tomatoes, onions, bell peppers, etc.

12. Butter!

13. Cheeses including feta cheese

14. Low-carb yogurts (check the labels). See Chapter Three to learn about great, **low-carb yogurt**!

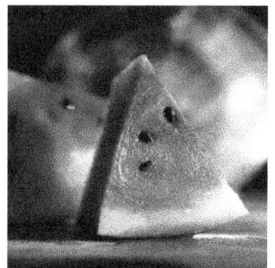 15. Melons including watermelon and honeydew melon

16. Low-carb flours including almond flour and coconut flour.

Note: See **Chapter Eleven** to learn about flours and breads.

17. Low-carb breads (either homemade or purchased)

18. Seeds including milled flax seed, chia seeds and sesame seeds

19. Olive oil and most vinegars

20. Stevia when a sugar substitute is required

D. The following high carb foods are avoided (This is not an exhaustive list, but – again – it is a good start):

1. Foods made from flours – like breads, pancakes, cakes, doughnuts, bagels, cookies, muffins, etc.

2. Sugars including corn syrup, honey and especially high fructose corn syrup

3. Milk

4. Starchy vegetables – like potatoes and corn

5. Rice

6. Most cereals (the carb counts are through the roof!)

7. Pasta

8. Non-berry, non-melon fruits

9. Soda pop and other soft beverages

10. Most "nutritional" shakes and protein drinks (check the carb count!)

> **E. Wonderful and delicious low-carb recipes are available in the** 1 To 5 Low-Carb Cooking **section of this book.**

I commend the recipes to you and invite you to try them out!

With these things in place, we add for emphasis:

Please Remember: This Is NOT A Diet (It Is A Feast!)

1. When we are hungry, we eat (with the above guidelines in mind).

2. We do NOT count calories (we count carbs and feast using the above guidelines).

III. Net Carb Count: A Deeper Understanding

1. Is the Carb Count of Foods Reduced When We ADD Fiber?

Many considering the low-carb regimen wonder if adding a high fiber food (such as chia seeds or hemp seeds) will reduce the net carb count of foods to which they are added.

The answer of course is "No." However, there is much more to this discussion – the idea of "absorbable" carbs is a critical concept: You will want to read on!

Each gram of fiber is first a gram of a subset (or, "kind") of carbohydrate. So, when you add fiber to a food, you also add a like amount to the total carb count of that food.

It is sad to say, but "one plus one plus one does NOT equal two!" Adding high fiber foods to a recipe does NOT reduce the net carb count of that recipe.

On the other hand, the added fiber may be beneficial to your diet in other ways!

2. Carb Counts and Grams per Ounce:

Carbohydrates in foods are customarily given in grams. For comparison (since most Americans are not as familiar with the metric system) there are approximately

84

28.35 grams per ounce when comparing mass. Mass is a measure of the total quantity – in our common experience we would think of this as "weight" (though – from a "technical" physics standpoint – weight depends on gravity) of the substance.

Be careful, here: Different foods have different densities – as a result, volumes will vary for the same weights. In other words, 80 grams (in weight of a food) is not necessarily ¼ cup in volume!

This becomes terribly important when you attempt to compare carb counts of foods. Variously, nutritional labels list a portion of the food in either teaspoons, tablespoons, ounces, quarter cups or grams (typically 80, 100 or more grams).

Keep in mind that in general: 3 teaspoons is 1 tablespoon, 2 tablespoons is one ounce, 8 ounces is one cup, 16 ounces is one pint, 32 ounces is one quart, 128 ounces is one gallon, etc.

You KNEW that math you learned in school was going to come in handy!

3. Minding Our Daily Carb Target:

It is also important to remember that the target for carbs under the Low-Carb Regimen is 60 to 80 grams of carbohydrates per day for those who are starting out, and an ongoing target of 50 grams of carbs per day for the long run.

4. Apples and Milk:

A single apple – depending on size and variety – has 26 grams of carbs. An eight ounce glass of milk (whether skim milk, 1% milk, 2% milk or whole milk) has 12 grams of carbs. Accordingly, most low-carb regimens seek to minimize intake of these foods. This also explains why those following the Low-Carb Regimen tend to substitute unsweetened almond milk and/or unsweetened coconut (my personal favourite!) milk into their eating regimens.

5. Carbs versus Net Carbs:

Total carbohydrate counts in foods are given on nutritional labels and then – depending on the food – additional sub-categories of carbohydrate may be given.

For instance, ¼ cup (80 grams for this product) of whole wheat flour has 21 grams of total carbohydrates. The 21 grams of total carbohydrates are made up of 4 grams of dietary fiber and 1 gram of sugars. The remaining 16 grams of carbohydrates – though not listed on the label – are starch.

In general, then, total carbohydrate count is given in three parts:

- Fiber (this is non-nutritional and is not normally absorbed in your metabolism)

- Sugars (obviously absorbed in a typical metabolism)

- Starch (also absorbed in a typical metabolism)

6. Quantity of "Absorbable" Carbs IS the Key:

Since the fiber amount of the carbohydrate is non-absorbable in a typical metabolism, then the part of the carbohydrate that is fiber DOES NOT COUNT for net carbohydrates.

If total carbs for a food is 16, but 11 of those carbs are fiber, then the net carb count is only 5 grams of carbohydrate.

7. The Starch and Sugar "Teeter-totter":

To make the long story short, vegetable carbohydrates allowed to naturally process over time tend to convert their sugars into starch.

A friend had a wonderful corn garden (In the Low-Carb Regimen we avoid corn and corn products now since these are high in absorbable carbohydrates). At that time, however, I knew nothing of the LCR and I was younger and even trimmer than I am now (I currently weigh what I did when I was twenty).

In fairness – from a mouth watering flavour perspective – there is something absolutely delectable about a fresh ear of corn, properly cooked, dripping in butter and lightly salted! Oh yeah – back yard barbecues of my "dietarily" wanton youth!

I didn't bring this up to create "an ear of corn craving," but to point out – as is commonly experienced – that the longer corn sits around after it is picked, the less sweet it tastes. The sugars of the corn – after picking – are naturally converted over time into starch.

When one (starch) goes up, the other (sugars) goes down: The starch and sugar teeter-totter. (The real trick here would be if you could get a vegetable that has transformed sugars into starch to reverse that process – kind of a vegetable anti-"aging" process.)

8. A Sound Replacement for that Buttered Ear of Corn:

In my home we love crunchy, flavourful stuff and – in honesty – yearn now and then for buttered popcorn or a buttered ear of corn. To reduce carbs, and yet keep that crunch and flavour, my wife found at Whole Foods:

Mother's brand Salted, Butter, Popcorn and Whole Grain Rice Cakes

Each cake does have 8 grams of total and net carbs (they are made with corn and with rice – two high carb foods we seek to minimize in our diet), so these cakes are NOT ultra low-carb foods.

On the other hand, they are a quick, easy, flavourful, filling, reasonably healthful food. In addition, they are great with almond butter!

9. The LCR:

Starches and sugars can have a big impact on other aspects of metabolism, but in the LCR generally the only concern is net carbohydrates.

This is one thing I personally like about the LCR: It is very simple!

Aim for a total of 50 grams of net carbs in your diet each day (60 to 80 grams of net carbs if you are just getting started).

Everything else, you can eat!

IV. Stimulating Our Bodies To Convert (Instead of Store) Fat:

1. As noted earlier in this chapter, the success of this process can be demonstrated by a simple, inexpensive test. See the **ketone testing** section of our current chapter for a review on verifying a fat "burning" metabolism.

2. As our bodies burn fat for energy, we tend to lose weight and begin to assume our appropriate body-mass appearance (not necessarily the unnatural and unhealthy appearance that some consider attractive).

3. When we feast using the LCR, energy levels and other bodily aspects may improve.

With the benefits of the LCR clearly in mind, we will want to:

V. Beware Hidden Carbs!

1. So, you're out to eat and you think to yourself, "onions are fine – I'll have onion rings." Wrong! The batter on those onion rings is loaded with carbs.

2. In another scenario, you hit your favourite fast food emporium and decide on chicken strips. Wrong! (Yep, the bread coating.)

3. Or you decide on chilli because it is high in fiber. Careful – those beans are loaded with carbs.

4. To make the long story short, if you are going to make this work, you must beware hidden carbs.

Chapter Four Conclusion:

In Chapter Four we explored the second of the Five LCR Steps: Activating a Fat-Burning Metabolism.

In upcoming chapters we will address the remaining three steps in our low-carb weight loss without dieting regimen:

- *Step Three: Optimizing Our Low-Carb Regimen,*

- *Step Four: Including Some Previously Excluded Foods, and*

- *Step Five: Maintaining Our Modified Low-Carb Regimen for a Lifetime.*

Up next: Step Three: Optimizing Our Low-Carb Regimen, Part I.

Chapter Five
Step Three - Optimization,
Part I:

Introduction:

Optimization is so broad a topic that it is presented here in two parts (each one a separate chapter). With this in mind we now consider Step Three: Optimization, Part I by looking at some factors that enable optimizing our low-carb regimen.

I. Step Three: Optimizing Our Low-Carb Regimen (LCR)

1. Personal Research

The human metabolism is a fascinating and varied piece of biochemical engineering!

It is abundantly clear from this diversity that variations in physiology, mentality, environment and emotional disposition create equally complex variations in optimizing our low-carb weight loss regimen.

The argument presented here, then, is that these factors need to be taken into consideration in order to produce a best case scenario for individual low-carb weight loss. Since one size does not fit all, in order to create optimization each of us needs to do our own "research" (frankly, trial and error) in order to find out what best "fine tunes" our own metabolism.

2. Five Areas to Refine in Our Regimen:

The refining process as already noted is really one of personal research and experimentation: Just what does work best for us as individuals?

Once we have discovered our optimization edge, then we can add or take away the "elements" of our success as we wish.

In consideration of this, five areas for refinement in our low-carb weight loss effort are:

> *a) Our Low-Carb Daily Regimen*
>
> *b) Our Low-Carb Regimen Variety*
>
> *c) Our Low-Carb Snack "Availability" Regimen*
>
> *d) Our Low-Carb Exercise Regimen*
>
> *e) Our Low-Carb Testing Regimen*

II. Our Low-Carb Daily Regimen

A comic character from my youth was renowned for his bottomless pit appetite. In one episode this character gave advice on how to get the most food on your plate at Thanksgiving. He suggested using a larger than average narrow rimmed plate to maximize the area where food could be piled without it appearing that we were taking more than our fellow diners!

1. The Great Secret

I bring this up to point out that by now we should be enjoying a new lifestyle of eating smaller, more delicious, more nutritious low-carb, high fat and high protein feasts. As a result of this process our stomachs have painlessly shrunk and it takes less to make us full.

There is a great secret here: We can – and should – eat less!

If you are not ready for this good news, go back to Step Two: Activating a Fat Burning Metabolism and continue with this process until you feel ready for Step Three.

2. Less More Frequently Really Is More

Less of the right low-carb foods is not only deliciously satisfying, but is also filling!

We no longer have to pack away gargantuan plates of high glycemic "junk" in order to meet the requirements of our appetite.

In this process, however, we must train our "eyes."

A little bit of food on a big plate tends to look too small. The same food, however, on a smaller plate looks abundant.

As a very serious proposal to optimizing our program: Start – if you have not already – using smaller plates!

It is a major lifestyle perspective change to realize that less of the right foods is more for your satisfaction and your overall well-being in life. We must put away the idea that we are going to lose a certain amount of weight and then go back to our old "carbaholic" ways.

If we fail to do this, we will fail in maintaining the gains of our new and vastly superior low-carb regimen.

3. Things to Do Daily

- Eat a small, nutritious low-carb "meal" every two to three hours:

  Do NOT skip meals!

- Eat (if only a packet of almonds) before you are truly hungry:

  Do NOT let yourself become truly hungry!

- Eat healthy proteins and fats:

  Do NOT skip proteins and fats!

- Eat healthy low-carb foods:

  Do NOT eat highly refined (high glycemic) high carb foods!

- Eat foods with known carb counts:

  Do NOT eat "hidden" carbs!

- Eat creatively delicious healthy low-carb foods:

  Do NOT become bored by always eating the same things!

- Eat to fuel your fat burning metabolism:

  Do NOT leave protein and fat "gaps" in your eating!

4. Protein in the Morning AND in the Evening

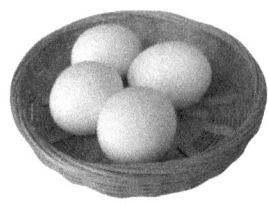 In this process a small quantity of protein before retiring for the evening is encouraged. A "big protein" (at least two eggs worth) breakfast is also suggested. Protein and fat throughout the day helps fuel your fat burning metabolism: Regularly add "wood" to the fat-burning "fire."

In all these things – if we have reached a plateau in our low-carb weight loss journey – a look at our daily low-carb regimen may reveal daily low-carb regimen areas that we can "optimize."

III. Our Low-Carb Regimen Variety

It's easy to get into a rut. After all, we can only eat so many almonds!

Here are some ideas on variety in our regimen:

1. Keeping Things Varied

For me assuring a consistent supply of quality fat and protein every few hours throughout my waking day is a key to optimization.

Of course, packets of dry roasted almonds, but also:

a) Hard boiled eggs:

By themselves the hard boiled eggs are great, but it takes very little to "devil" them deliciously: See the recipe in the **1 To 5 Low-Carb Cooking Guide** at the end of this book.

b) Left over chicken, beef, pork or lamb:

Low-Carb dinner foods left over and served cold or hot make great additional meals!

c) Peanut butter protein balls:

See the recipe in the **1 To 5 Low-Carb Cooking Guide** and consider adding the bakers cocoa. When you do, they come out like an unbelievably good for you Reese's Peanut Butter Cup (Out of country readers: This is a popular candy bar in America).

d) Whey shakes:

Check the net carbs per the labels and select truly low-carb brands of whey! You will discover that chocolate, vanilla and strawberry are readily available. In addition, one can add almost any low-carb flavor, low-carb fruit or low-carb, CarbMaster yogurt. Or make them overwhelmingly creamy by using unsweetened, unflavored coconut milk for your fluid base: Do NOT use fruit juices (much too high in carbohydrates)! Also, avoid off-the-shelf "protein shakes" – most of these are high carb. Low-carb exceptions include: Atkins Advantage Protein Shakes and 100 Calorie Muscle Milk Shakes (Cytosports' vanilla 100 calorie shake is lower carb than its chocolate version).

Note: According to its labelling, EAS markets a relatively low-carb protein shake. However, there appears to be a component in this shake that – for me – interferes with my low-carb regimen. Accordingly, I do not use this product. *We are each – obviously – unique. It is essential in the LCR to note carefully those foods which best work (and which do NOT work) for you!*

e) Celery sticks with cheese, cream cheese:

I like to press a few blueberries into the cream cheese "log." For variety I fill the celery with peanut or almond butter (but don't use raisins – way too high carb!).

f) Pumpkin protein slices:

See the recipe in the **1 To 5 Low-Carb Cooking Guide**. Avoid store bought "protein bars" – almost all are high carb.

g) Precooked bacon strips:

Yep, protein and fat – just what the low-carb regimen doctor ordered! I love to have them with slices of pepper jack cheese.

h) Pre-prepared salad:

We like Romaine lettuce, cucumbers, bell peppers, spinach, watercress, avocado, sliced strawberries, and freshly ground pepper with olive oil and red wine vinegar! I like to crown mine with some feta or Parmesan cheese. Avoid creamy, high carb dressings!

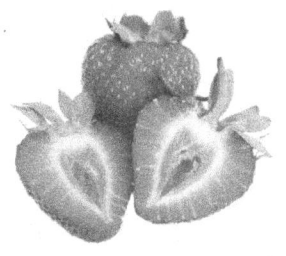

i) A small dish of berries:

Try adding either whipping cream (many are low-carb, but check the labels) or topping with non-whipped, heavy whipping cream, half and half cream or unsweetened, unflavored coconut milk.

j) Low-carb (made with Splenda) jello:

Top it with some low-carb whipped topping! It is really good!

k) A SINGLE Minnie Beasley Almond Lace cookie:

They are not sufficiently low-carb to eat more than one for a snack, but they are a great treat!

l) A latte made with unsweetened, unflavored coconut milk:

For variety – and rich flavour – add a tablespoon of low-carb whipped cream topping, non-whipped heavy whipping cream or half and half cream!

m) Toasted sesame seaweed snacks:

You really have to try these – they are delicious, nutritious and taste very much like kettle corn!

n) Bell pepper strips:

Crisp, delicious and a great snack with or without a low-carb dip!

Now if – with all of these wonderful, ready to go, quick and easy snacks – you cannot satisfy your appetite and instead feel the need to munch some high glycemic "food," then you should consider returning to Chapter Three and overcoming your carb cravings!

If you are thinking: These are great snacks, how about some meals, then check out:

The LCR approach to food preparation, see the **1 To 5 Low-Carb Cooking Guide** at the end of this book.

2. Finding Our Plateaus

Once ketosis is established, the obese pounds of weight loss tend to shed readily. On the other hand – for many – once the obese pounds are lost, getting our bodies to lose the remaining ten to twenty pounds of weight that comprise the "overweight" range of the Body Mass Index (BMI) can be a significant hurdle (especially those final ten pounds before arriving at our BMI "ideal" weight).

Overcoming our plateaus is really what Step Three: Optimization is all about. Use the ideas contained in this Chapter, Part I (the section you are currently reading) and Part II (our upcoming **Chapter Six**) in order to gain success in shedding those more difficult last few pounds.

Keep in mind, also, that even though these pounds tend to shed much more slowly, they still tend to respond to adherence to a low-carb regimen lifestyle.

Be prepared to "keep on keeping on" and plan to persevere. As you stay the course – eating low-carb, fuelling your fat burning metabolism with appropriate protein and fat intake, and utilizing light aerobic exercise at least once (and preferably two or three times) each day – you should discover the success you seek.

IV. Our Low-Carb Snack "Availability" Regimen

When it comes to low-carb "snacking" (a snack is really just a small meal!), failure to prepare is preparing to fail.

In this it would seem that most of us are looking for a "magic bullet" when It comes to low-carb snacking: We want food that is appealing, delicious, easy (to obtain, to store and to ingest in a convenient and non-messy fashion) and relatively inexpensive.

Many "low-carbers" spend times searching for truly low-carb protein bars (16 grams of net carbs per bar tends to be the best you'll find). I think a better approach is to invest in a soft (collapsible), personal sized food cooler (one big enough to carry snacks with you while you travel and when you are at work).

- Coleman 9-Can Soft Cooler with Liner for $9.88 with hard plastic interior liner

- Coleman 9-Can Soft Cooler with Collapsible Liner for $10.50

- Coleman Blue Ice Soft Pack for under two dollars

- Rubbermaid Blue Ice Mini Pack for several dollars

I like to freeze the blue ice pack and have my snacks in "ready to go" containers in my refrigerator. When morning arrives I simply load the frozen blue ice and the cooled snack containers into the collapsible personal cooler and then take it with me to work. These foods are then readily available whenever I want them.

They are also available to eat while I commute, but – a caution here – do NOT drive distracted (even by great low-carb snacks)!

For great foods to put in your cooler, again, see the snack foods listed above in:

III. Our Low-Carb Regimen - 1. Keeping Things Varied

Chapter Five Conclusion:

We have yet to look at "Our Low-Carb Exercise" and "Our Low-Carb Testing." Conveniently, this is the topic of our next chapter, Chapter Six – Step Three: Optimization, Part II.

Chapter Six

Step Three - Optimization, Part II:

Be the Low-carb "All You Can Be"

Introduction:

*In our previous chapter, **Step Three: Optimization – Part I**, as well as in other earlier chapters in this book we looked at the requisite background information needed to embrace the ideas contained in the subject at hand: Step Three - Optimization, Part II. Please keep in mind: The current information requires that which went before.*

Got Vitamin D?

Since many of us have eliminated dairy milk from our diet (much too high carb!), we are missing Vitamin D supplementation (dairy milk is normally Vitamin D enriched).

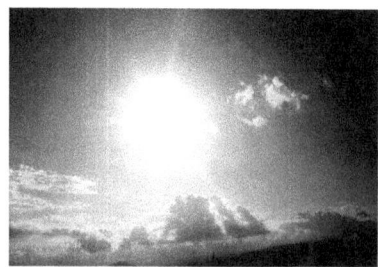 Accordingly, we will need to either ensure sufficient daily skin exposure to the sun through our outdoor activities so that we can produce the required Vitamin D, or we will

need to add Vitamin D supplements to our diet. Insufficient daily Vitamin D can interfere with healthful metabolism and low-carb weight loss.

V. Our Low-Carb Exercise

The caution here – of course – is NOT to overdo the exercise and thereby "kick" our metabolisms out of a fat burning (ketosis) energy cycle. If we stop producing ketones (noticeably present in urine, in breath and testable per the **ReliOn Ketone test strips**), then we should suspect that our exercise level is too high for an effective low-carb regimen.

Another indicator that we may have derailed our fat-burning process is – if there are no changes in our regimen other than increased exercise – that our weight either "tables" (a plateau in which our weight remains static) or that we begin to gain weight. Keep in mind the greater density of muscle compared to fat and measure changes not only in weight but also in the inches that measure portions of your body (biometric measurements). Again, it may be necessary to choose between low-carb regimen weight loss and expanded muscle development: The two do not usually go hand in hand!

1. Light Aerobic Exercise

While heavy exercise can interfere with our fat-burning metabolism, ten to fifteen minutes of light aerobic exercise before breakfast helps set our metabolisms for the "big protein" breakfast that we will consume. This can also be a convenient and consistent time for biometric measurement of our progress. Remember: Failure to plan is planning to fail.

I find the use of my Wii exercise software useful and convenient for this purpose.

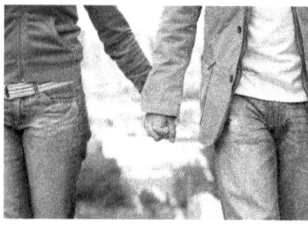 Those who find it practical might enjoy a walk, a relaxing bicycle ride, a light run, skipping rope, a swim if you have a pool, some aerobic "stepping," a little tennis, some "hoops," some "dancercise," some light callisthenics – the list goes on and on: You get the idea!

Via Steps **One** and **Two** as described in our previous chapters we have lost our "obese" pounds and are now working on the ten to twenty pounds that keep us in the "overweight" category per the BMI (Body Mass Index). If you are not at this point in your program, please return to Steps One and Two as needed. The important thing is to regularly incorporate light aerobic exercise into your daily regimen at least once – and if possible – two or three times each day.

Of course, a regular waking and sleeping time is essential to success in this effort. Here also is an area that can impact the success (or failure) of our low-carb weight loss effort.

2. Sleep and Weight Loss:

In a sense sleep is "resting exercise." At the very least, physical exercise – not to mention optimal mental performance – is less likely to be viable without sufficient rest.

More to the point of this chapter, quality of sleep may impact low-carb weight loss efficiency

Adequate sleep is also essential for healing and for growth. In spite of significant research, however, much remains unknown regarding the mental and physiologic processes of sleep. It appears that the brain cycles through phases – delineated by the kind, quality and duration of brain waves – during sleep. These phases appear to allow the processing, incorporation and filing of short term memory and experiences into long term memory. This process is demonstrated to increase memory recall in testing situations (don't stay up all night "cramming"). In addition, "sleeping on it" appears to provide "perspective" benefits in conflict resolution. All of these aspects of adequate sleep may then provide benefit to our low-carb weight loss effort.

The holy grail in sleep phases is thought to be REM (Rapid Eye Movement) sleep. During this phase dreaming occurs and it may be that REM sleep is a key to improved biologic performance. If this is true, then adequate REM sleep – a possible mental and physiologic "housekeeping" process – may play a particularly vital role in low-carb weight loss.

A useful analogy to the maintenance process of the adequate sleep requirement is found in computer science.

Early computers required "housekeeping" processes that re-arranged files in order to optimize retrieval and maximize storage efficiency. While this is mostly automatic today, computers still require disk defragmentation for peak performance. Also common in Windows based systems is the need to "clean the registry." Our brains as "biologic computers" appear to perform similar functions thru adequate sleep.

As noted before, our bodies repair themselves and grow during adequate sleep. We used to tell our kids that in order to reach their maximum height they needed more sleep. Teens today average less than six hours of sleep (frequently, much less than six hours) on school nights. As a teacher of students learning secondary Math content I can verify that this is insufficient for optimal performance in the classroom.

Regarding growing while sleeping, the ongoing increase in generational height appears, then, to be more linked to nutritional changes and genetic selection over the decades than to sufficiency of sleep. In this, height may be desirable for other reasons than just vanity. For instance, life success is frequently associated with height as in the case of political elections. There is some research to suggest that – all things being equal – the taller candidate tends to win.

3. Stress and weight loss:

Stress works against productive low-carb weight loss function.

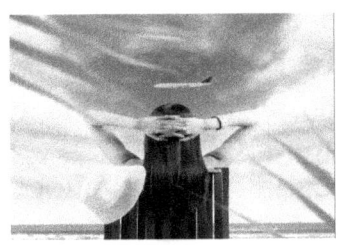 Among other things, stress can increase insulin production. This is a particularly serious problem for health and weight loss in those of us who are insulin resistant. See the section of this book on **How to Know If You Are Insulin Resistant**.

Dealing with stress is so much a problem that treating stress disorders has become a major issue in America. If you'll allow the "tongue in cheek" observation: Since most Americans are overweight or obese, at the very least we can stress about our weight!

Among methods for dealing with stress is the protocol known as humour therapy.

4. Laughter and "thumping" your thalamus:

Many of us truly appreciate being around those who laugh heartily.

Laughing regularly – not like a lunatic, but a hearty belly laugh – produces numerous health benefits including stress reduction. In addition a good belly laugh has been likened by some to a healthy "thumping" of the thalamus.

Health and Nursing Issues Australia notes that according to WebMD 2003:

A study in Japan shows that laughter lowers blood sugar after a meal. Keiko Hayashi, Ph.D., R.N, of the University of Tsukuba in Ibaraki, Japan, and his team performed a study of 19 people with type 2 diabetes.

They collected the patients' blood before and two hours after a meal. The patients attended a boring 40 minute lecture after dinner on the first night of the study. On the second night, the patients attended a 40 minute comedy show. The patients' blood sugar went up after the comedy show, but much less than it did after the lecture. The study found that even when patients without diabetes did the same testing, a similar result was found. Scientists concluded that laughter is good for people with diabetes. They suggest that chemical messengers made during laughter may help the body compensate for the disease.

To really understand our metabolisms, then, adequate information is required. One way to obtain this information is from a variety of available home testing approaches.

VI. Our Low-carb Testing

1. Simple Biometrics

In my personal optimization process, simple biometrics appear sufficient for fine tuning my regimen. Again, however, others may desire greater precision.

2. How Can We Be More Precise?

We can tweak our low-carb weight loss regimen by keeping all things in our regimen consistent, modifying just one thing in our regimen (such as trying a new food), and then measuring the results.

In this "vein" (pun intended! – since blood testing may be required), we can know with relative ease the precise changes in our basic blood chemistry. If we see the result as an improvement, then we may wish to incorporate "the change" into our daily regimen.

The converse would also be true.

3. Time to use the glycemic index

The concept of the glycemic index may be of use in this process. In general, however, it has been sufficient for me to recognize and eliminate highly refined high carb foods. Unless foods are specifically prepared – normally by me – to be low-carb, I avoid them. I especially avoid pastas, breads, cupcakes, brownies, pancakes, syrups, sugars, cakes, cheesecakes, icings, pies, candies, ice creams, and other highly refined high carb store bought foods.

On the other hand, I eat liberally of any of the above when they are homemade and truly low-carb.

Note: I have found that there is no low-carb version for a "true" pasta. Although there are "kinda sorta" pastas made from strips of plant products, true pastas are ALL high carb. There are low-carb versions, however, of the other "food" items listed above.

So, how can we really know what impact such foods have on our chemistries?

4. Home Testing

Note: To bypass the information on "Home Testing" and proceed to the next section, please go to "Hard-Boiled Thoughts".

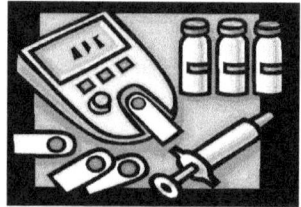 A raft of simple and convenient "test yourself at home" kits are available to measure blood glucose. Less are available to measure cholesterol, and I found only one relatively inexpensive package that would measure blood lipids including triglycerides, HDL and LDL.

Although these home test kits normally are intended for those dealing with diabetes or elevated cholesterol levels, they may be useful in getting an accurate understanding of some of our individual chemistries. Along these lines, blood glucose is a measure of blood sugar and is of particular interest for the insulin resistant. As observed earlier in this book, insulin is produced to transport glucose in the bloodstream to our cells for use as energy. The insulin resistant tend to store this "rejected" glucose as fat throughout the body and particularly as belly fat: See the section of this book on "How to Know If You Are Insulin Resistant."

5. Interpreting Blood Test Results

In order to do home testing, you will need to order the relevant kits and also be willing to subject yourself – as many in our population do daily – to a finger or arm prick that will allow a small sample of blood. Hygiene is key, or course, when piercing the epidermal layer and antibacterial protections should be applied. In addition, those suffering from HIV or other blood transmitted pathogens should avoid taking blood samples unless instructed to do so by their physician.

For those who are testing, once the drop of blood is collected it is then introduced to the appropriate test strip for absorption. The test strip is then either compared to a colour coded chart (a rather subjective process) or read by a meter (a more objective process).

Note: Blood test ranges:

Most sources of information on "normal" body chemistry values emphasize that the ability of a properly trained medical professional is key to interpreting and using such results. Keep this in mind if you elect to test at home.

Having said this, the above link provides some "normal" ranges.

6. Blood Testing

Much in the way of home blood testing kits is specifically for those who are monitoring – under a doctor's supervision – blood sugar. Typically, these individuals do so under a diagnosis or suspicion of diabetes.

With this in mind, here are some of the available home test kits with links to where they can be obtained:

Simple glucose tests – Blood glucose
kits **as well as a** home administered A1c:

The A1c gives an "average" picture of glucose levels over recent weeks. Typical glucometers give a "snapshot" of blood sugar levels at the time of testing. The glucometric test kits, then, are the ones that will provide information on how a specific food impacts our blood sugar levels.

These kits range from around thirty dollars to as much as a few hundred dollars. Here are a couple of more readily available home testing kits.

- **ReliOn Blood Glucose Meter** with Test Strips

- **Bayer Blood Glucose Test System**

- The **CardioChek PA meter** is popular for measuring cholesterol and triglycerides.

- **Simple cholesterol tests**

- **Simple lipid tests**

So what could we do with the information gleaned from these home testing kits?

As noted before, the impact of specific foods on our blood chemistry could be of use in "fine tuning" our dietary regimen. Low-carb weight loss theory suggests that our low-carb, high fat, high protein regimen should reduce blood sugar and cholesterol levels while providing improvement in overall lipid levels. We typically desire higher HDL measurements and lower LDL measurements.

7. Understanding Blood Lipids

According to wiseGeek:

a) Lipids

The three major purposes of lipids in the body are storing energy, aiding the development of cell membranes and serving as components of hormones and vitamins. In healthcare, physicians order lipid tests or lipid profiles to measure cholesterol and triglycerides in a person's blood. "Lipoprotein" is the medical term used to refer to a combination of fat and protein.

b) Cholesterol

Cholesterol is a naturally occurring substance in the body and is comprised of lipids. It is separated into two types: high-density lipoprotein (HDL) and low-density lipoprotein (LDL). HDL is often referred to as "good cholesterol" because it is beneficial to a person's health. LDL is often called "bad cholesterol" because too much of it can be harmful.

c) Triglycerides

Triglycerides are the chemical formation of animal and vegetable fats. In molecular form, three molecules of fatty acids combine with glycerol to form triglycerides. In the human body, these are carried through the blood plasma, and unused molecules are stored in the body as fat.

Triglycerides provide twice [the energy to the body that carbohydrates do].

Triglycerides are not only present in the body through the consumption of fats, but also through the consumption of carbohydrates. Most carbohydrates are naturally turned into triglycerides by the body. Therefore, a diet low in fat, but high in carbohydrates, may serve to increase triglyceride levels.

A low-carbohydrate diet often helps to lower triglyceride levels.

8. Urine Testing

In Chapter **Four** we looked at the simple process of **testing for a fat burning metabolism** (ketosis) through the use of easily obtained and inexpensive Ketone test strips:

A more comprehensive approach that includes glucose measurements along with lipid testing is available. See: **Urine glucose/ketone plus** testing.

VII. "Hard Boiled" Thoughts:

In homage to the hard-boiled eggs discussed in **Step Three: Optimization, Part I**, here are some "hard-boiled" thoughts:

In life we tend to do what we really want to do. Lots of people want to lose weight, but they actually really want to continue their "carbaholic" eating of "foods" that work against their weight loss goals.

Many want to be fit but are unwilling to engage in the appropriate exercises that support this goal.

If we really want to lose weight – in most cases – we can. Those who are diligent in applying the appropriate low-carb weight loss steps should find success. Those who are diligent and yet do not succeed will want to seek appropriate medically trained support.

As you choose what you really want, I wish you success in your low-carb weight loss regimen!

Chapter Seven

Step Four - Including:

Adding Back Select Previously Excluded Foods

In order to establish our weight-loss without dieting (fat-burning) metabolism, we scrupulously eliminated all high carb foods. This was necessary in order to overcome carb withdrawal, to activate our fat-burning metabolism and to optimize our low-carb weight-loss without dieting regimen. Having established a successful pattern in our low-carb "way of life," we now look at Step Four of the five steps of the LCR. In this step we will optimize our low-carb nutrition by adding back select higher (but NOT high-glycemic) carb foods.

Again, the Five Steps of the LCR are:

One: Overcoming Carb Withdrawal

Two: Activating a Fat Burning Metabolism

Three: Optimizing Our Low-Carb Regimen

Four: Including Select Previously Excluded Foods

Five: Maintaining Our LCR for a Lifetime

I. Recent JAMA Articles

Those following the "low-carb" news may have noted recent JAMA (Journal of the American Medical Association) verifications of the efficacy of the low-carb, high protein, high healthful fat eating regimen.

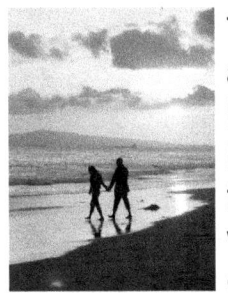 The above referenced **JAMA article** observes that REE (Resting Energy Expenditures) and TEE (Total Energy Expenditures) were least affected following weight loss by those whose weight loss resulted from a low-carb eating regimen. The significance of this is its impact on weight gain following weight loss. The synopsis of the article states that:

". . . reduced energy expenditure following weight loss is thought to contribute to weight gain."

Another **JAMA article** comparing several weight loss approaches (the Low-Carb Eating Regimen is a dramatic refinement of Atkins concepts based on the foundation of dealing with insulin resistance) offered the following conclusion:

"In this study, premenopausal overweight and obese women assigned to follow the Atkins diet, which had the lowest carbohydrate intake, lost more weight and experienced more favourable overall metabolic effects at 12 months than women assigned to follow the Zone, Ornish, or LEARN diets. While questions remain about

long-term effects and mechanisms, a low-carbohydrate, high-protein, high-fat diet may be considered a feasible alternative recommendation for weight loss."

II. Perspective on Steps One Through Three

With positive JAMA support in mind, let us put our low-carb eating regimen steps into perspective:

- Steps One and Two should allow us to shed our "obese" pounds (those pounds associated with obese weight ranges per the **BMI Body Mass Index**).

- In Step Three we began the generally more gradual process of establishing success in losing the top half of the BMI's "overweight" pounds for our sex/body-build/height classification.

- In Step Four we focus on the remaining half of our BMI classification "overweight" pounds.

III. As We Add Back Selected Foods, We Must Avoid Eating Like Carbaholics

It is fascinating to encounter those whose mentality is:

"I don't like – and will not eat – non-starchy vegetables."

In my thinking what people who consciously choose to be carbaholics are saying is:

"I am addicted to carbohydrates AND I love my addiction."

1. Their first need – of course – is to recognize that carbaholism is an addiction.

One could picture a group meeting:

"Hello, my name is _____ (fill in the name here), and I'm a carbaholic."

2. The second need of the carbaholic is to gain the required knowledge about carbohydrate addiction and the dangers of insulin resistance.

Insulin Resistance is a pre-diabetic condition that may affect or through the course of their lifetimes may affect a majority of people in America. From these two needs comes the opportunity to make an informed decision to change from carbaholism to the healthy and enjoyable LCR.

3. The third need of the carbaholic is to begin to experience real food flavour.

It usually shocks the confirmed carbaholic, but they may discover – once they stop inundating their taste buds with highly-refined, high carb "foods" – that the healthful low-carb, high protein, high healthful fat foods they are currently avoiding are more delicious than they – in their carbaholic addiction – can imagine.

4. The fourth need of the carbaholic is to make an informed choice.

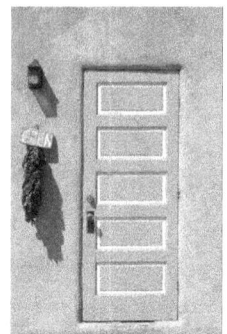 It is as if there is a door before us. When we open the door of healthful low-carb, high protein, high healthful fat eating we can enter into a life of increased health, vigor and vitality. Once one has passed through this door flavours may explode in delightful ways not previously imagined. Being truly hungry can become a thing of the past (in the low-carb eating regimen we do not diet, we feast! AND we do NOT allow ourselves to become truly hungry). In this process we replace carbaholism and dieting with a "low-carb, high protein, high healthy fat" renewed capacity for fulfilled living which may then become our norm.

In contrast to these benefits we can refuse to open the door to the healthful low-carb, high protein, high healthful fat eating regimen. We can choose to remain addicted to carbohydrates and increase our risk to the myriad health problems associated with the carbaholic lifestyle.

IV. Rates of Weight Loss

Rates of weight loss are obviously a unique experience for each of us. It does seem to be true, however, that the obese pounds – once a fat burning (ketosis) metabolism is established – shed more quickly than the "merely" overweight pounds of the **BMI scale**.

In my experience it took about eight months to shed the 40 obese pounds with which I began. It has taken about six to eight weeks to shed each of the remaining groups of five pounds that make up the "overweight" portion of the BMI scale.

V. Adding Back Previously Excluded Foods

When it comes to adding back foods (previously excluded in Steps One thru Three) into our eating regime **low glycemic**, high fiber carbohydrates become the most obvious candidates.

Using the "trial and error" and body chemistry methods described in the two chapters comprising Step Three: Optimizing Our Low-Carb Regimen, we add back selected foods to our diet. Careful attention to biometrics and our sense of well-being allow us to identify foods, portions and timings in eating those foods that support our efforts.

In a sense, then, we are revisiting the question posed in the chapter, "So, Where's My Bread?"

We now refine the answer contained in that chapter based on the successful completion of The Five Steps in our Low-Carb Regimen. As noted above, we are now adding back low glycemic legumes and selected relatively low-carb whole grains IF our individual metabolisms demonstrate success when they are eaten.

One size definitely does not fit all in this process.

Insulin resistance is a complex issue and produces diverse needs based on our unique metabolic requirements. Per our discussion in Step Three, medically interpreted body chemistry results may be called for depending on your individual needs.

1. Relatively Low-carb Whole Grain Cereals

Natures Path (also available in limited selections through Walmart) markets a relatively low-carb, high fiber **SmartBran cereal**.

At 11 net grams of carbs (after subtracting the fiber) per half cup portion, this is much lower than most cereals whose carb counts are 30 to 50 grams of carbs per serving.

In addition, Bob's Red Mill markets an organic, high fiber **Hot Cereal** with flaxseed with a net carb count of 17 grams per one third cup serving. In particular, I have found this cereal useful to add a "rustic grain" flavour and texture in my low-carb bread recipes.

2. Relatively Low-Carb Legumes

Following the philosophy of the low glycemic index, beans and other legumes (such as lentils and peas) – although higher in carbohydrate – may be low in blood sugar impact. The argument is that the starch in many legumes consists of types that, in most people, are either digested slowly or not digested in the small intestine at all (resistant starch).

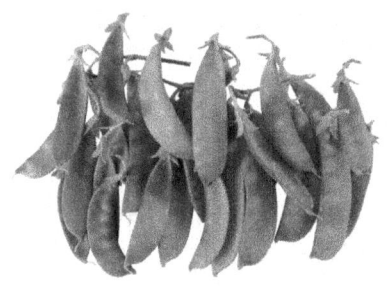

Therefore, in moderation, legumes may have a small glycemic impact.

The key here, however, is moderation. As noted above, our unique tolerances regarding legumes vary with the diversity of our metabolisms. Trial and error, metabolic testing and attention to our personal "well being" indicators will provide the necessary guidance to how legumes may best be incorporated into our eating regimens.

3. Atkins Advantage Vanilla Nutrition Shake

After looking at countless "health" shakes, it is nice to finally find one that is low-carb and high protein. There are four individual 11 ounce containers in the four container carton sold by Walmart.

Walmart customer reviews vary regarding this product with several stating that they prefer the flavour of other "nutrition" shakes. From the perspective of low-carb eating these "complaints" miss the point: The Atkins Vanilla Nutrition Shake is nutritious, relatively high protein and only 1 net gram of carbs (after subtracting the fiber) per an 11 ounce container.

Those recommending other "shakes" (such as EAS) may be promoting 30 to 40 grams (or more) of carbs per container beverages! I have found an EAS shake whose label states that it is low-carb. However – for me

– the EAS low-carb version behaved very much like a high carb beverage.

The Atkins Advantage Nutrition Shake comes in Vanilla (my favourite), Dark Chocolate, Mocha, Berry and Strawberry. However, there are variations in net carb counts. The non-Vanilla flavours have slightly higher carb counts.

The walmart.com website states regarding this product:

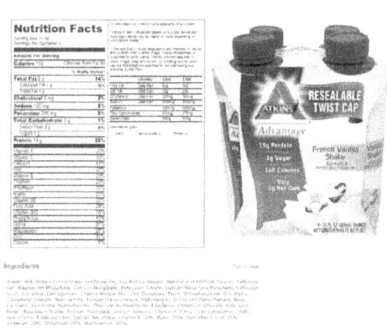

The Atkins Advantage Vanilla Shake is a powerful ingredient for a successful weight loss and weight management. Smooth, tasty and yummy, each serving contains a single gram of net carbs. The Atkins vanilla shake offers a low-sugar mix of high-quality protein, fiber, vitamins, and minerals. You will love the rich texture of this weight loss nutrition shake. Available in a four-pack, the Atkins Advantage shakes are a convenient and affordable option for weight management.

The website claims that the Atkins Advantage Vanilla Shake is:

- Delicious
- A Low-Sugar Mix
- Weight Loss and Weight Management

4. Countless Other Moderately Low-Carb Foods To Consider Adding Back

Check the glycemic index and read the labels for carb counts of perspective foods. By Step Four we are ready to expand our previously limited – only very low-carb – food selections. As per above, at this stage many look again at the moderately low-carb legumes.

Pay attention, however, to the impact of each added back food. This is to say that it is wiser to add back a single new food at a time and observe how this impacts our fat-burning metabolisms, our well-being and our weight.

Obviously, we will keep the foods that work for us and exclude the others!

VI. Adding Back Heavier Exercise

Once the obese pounds are shed heavier exercise becomes more viable. This process depends on one's individual metabolism and is unique to each individual. The concern is that heavier exercises might cause an individual's "fuel" process to "come out" of the fat-burning (ketosis) metabolism. On the other hand, heavier exercises tend to replace fat with muscle (which most see as desirable).

Heavier Exercise: The Gold's XRS 30 Home Gym

In this – as noted in previous chapters – it is key to keep in mind that the greater density of muscle can result in less weight loss or even in weight gains.

Walmart markets an inexpensive, low-end home gym that may be of use in this process. At under two hundred dollars, for my relatively modest needs, the**Gold's XRS 30 Home Gym** is proving invaluable.

The Walmart description states:

Build incredible total-body strength with the Gold's Gym XRS 30 System. Featuring a 112 lb. weight stack, this Gold's Gym home gym delivers a full-range of workout options and up to 300 lbs. of resistance for maximum results. Plus, with Gold's Gym XRS 30's combination chest press/fly station, you'll get twice the upper-body results. This home gym also features a 4-roll leg developer, high and low pulleys, a lat bar and an exercise chart designed by a Certified Personal Trainer.

If you're a fan of "preacher curls," a separate add on allows this option.

Those interested in the XRS 30 should keep in mind that it takes several hours of patient effort in order to assemble. In addition, the shipping weight makes it more affordable to arrange for the free "site to store" shipping. If you transport the gym in a smaller vehicle, opening the heavy shipping container and "breaking the gym down" into easier to carry portions may be a good option.

Choices Regarding Too Much Exercise

It feels so good (all those endorphins) to "pump iron" and make muscles bulge.

However, a choice may have to be made here. Are you really willing to give up a fat-burning metabolism in order to bulk out with muscles (a simple ketone test strip will indicate your ketone level). You may be (in which case you will not be concerned as the scale shows your weight going up).

On the other hand – in order to maintain a fat-burning metabolism – you may need to go easy on the heavier exercise.

Chapter Seven Conclusion:

Four steps to success in our low-carb eating regimen are now complete!

At this stage in my personal experience I was at fifty-three pounds lost with a mere ten pounds remaining until reaching the desired non-overweight status.

In accordance with the slower, more deliberate weight loss typical as these last pounds are shed, these final ten pounds could take about three to four more months of utterly enjoyable low-carb, high protein, high healthful fat feasting.

At that time the final step (Step Five: Maintaining the Low-Carb Regimen for a Lifetime) becomes the focal point.

In the meantime, the low-carb eating regimen allows me to eat whenever I am hungry and is so much more enjoyable, healthful and beneficial than other methods that I have experienced. In addition, it is an absolute delight to get back to heavier exercise along with the ongoing light aerobic workouts!

Those as diligent in following this approach may experience similar results. In all of this I wish you success in your own low-carb eating regimen!

Next up: Chapter Eight - Step Five: Maintaining Our Low-Carb Regimen for a Lifetime!

Chapter Eight

Step Five - Maintaining:
Our LCR Lifestyle

"Step Five: Maintaining the LCR" is a "rest of our lives" pursuit. As such it is a joyous growth of low-carb vitality and weight-maintenance without dieting.

Included in "Chapter Eight - Maintaining" is:

I. A description of "counter-intuitives"

II. A discussion of overcoming obstacles in the LCR

III. A commentary on the low-carb process

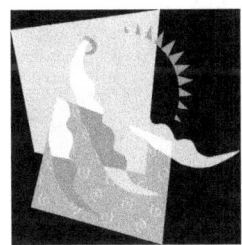

1. What a delight

2. Goal reached

3. Low-carb eating regimen versus "traditional" weight loss

4. Removing the "hunger barrier" by changing what you eat

5. Overcoming insulin resistance and discovering flavour

6. A beautiful secret

Keeping the above "map" in mind, we now look at "counter-intuitives" – those LCR precepts that may be in opposition to commonly held concepts regarding weight loss.

I. Counter-Intuitives: A Reminder To Keep Doing The Right Things

Our regimen began with the explicit understanding that the LCR is for those healthy enough to undertake it.

We emphasized that those under medical care, or needing medical care, will – of course – follow the counsel of the appropriately trained medical professionals to whom they have entrusted their health.

With this caveat in mind, we now note that succeeding at the low-carb regimen requires setting aside certain preconceived, supposedly "common sense" ideas.

For emphasis: *All of the "concepts" listed below presume the adoption of the LCR as detailed in this book.*

1. We must eat in order to lose weight

This implies that we are eating appropriately according to the low-carb regimen!

Specifically, we must eat low-carb, high healthful fat, high protein foods while avoiding high carb, low fat, low protein foods!

2. We must eat fat to keep our bodies from storing fat

This implies that healthful fat is our friend!

3. We must avoid allowing ourselves to become truly hungry

Since going truly hungry puts our metabolisms into "starvation mode" (which shuts down our fat burning metabolism), we eat more frequent meals – essentially "pre-eating" before we eat our more formal meals.

We eat until we are satisfied, not until we are stuffed – if we are still hungry 20 minutes after eating reasonable portions, we can always eat more at that time.

Over time (as we adapt to the Low-Carb Regimen) we eat smaller, more frequent meals rather than larger, less frequent meals

We can eat "whatever we want, whenever we want" as long as it is low-carb, high healthful fat and high protein: Point in case, if I feel a hunger pang, I eat a snack pack of toasted almonds, a couple of strips of bacon, some cheddar cheese, some hard-boiled eggs (I like mine **deviled, low-carb**), or some leftover low-carb foods that are on hand.

4. We must avoid strenuous exercise in order to maintain a fat-burning metabolism.

Light aerobic exercise (a ten to twenty minute walk) one to three times per day supports a fat-burning metabolism while heavy and/or strenuous exercise thwarts a fat-burning metabolism.

Note: While butter, cheese and cream cheese are low-carb, ALL dairy milk – regardless of fat content – is high carb. When in doubt, read the labels!

II. Overcoming Obstacles in the LCR: Staying With Our Counter-Intuitives

1. From Where Have We Come?

It is absolutely possible to make a mess out of the LCR and thereby obtain disastrous results. My point is that success in the LCR is a bit like the admonition: "Do or do NOT – there is no try."

Of course, all human processes are made up of a series of starts and re-starts. None of us is perfect in our performance.

The success of this program in my personal weight loss has very little to do with any native discipline on my part (frankly, I have very little!) and everything to do with how easy it is to eat according to LCR guidelines once these are known and understood.

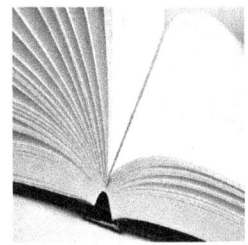 The point here, however, is that those seeking to adopt the LCR need to actually know, understand and implement the concepts (as opposed to trying to adopt only parts of the Low-Carb Regimen).

2. Half-Hearted Low-Carb Regimen Efforts:

For those of us who have enjoyed Disney's Pirates of the Caribbean theme ride, "partial" low-carb efforts are like the pirate with one foot on the dock and one foot in the boat: As he straddles half way between the two, you know he is headed for disaster!

3. It Doesn't Work If You Don't Work It:

It always amazes me to be around those seeking to follow a low-carb regimen who knowingly violate major precepts of the regimen and then are disappointed when they do not make progress in their weight-loss goals. It is a bit like repeating our mistakes over and over, but – each time the mistake is repeated – somehow expecting a different result!

For most, a fat-burning metabolism is a finely tuned metabolic mechanism. Just think how much it took to get the keto-lipolytic (fat-burning) process going.

Along with this, keep in mind that the LCR does not work if you don't work it.

4. One Foot on the Gas with One Foot on the Brake:

A different eating regimen is required for those who wish to exercise strenuously. Trying to eat low-carb while undertaking strenuous exercise is like trying to drive a car with one foot fully on the gas pedal and the other foot fully on the brake. Whether the car moves or not, the wear and tear are likely to be devastating to the car's systems.

5. Strenuous Exercise and Binging Shut Down a Fat-Burning Metabolism:

Many really like the physical (endorphin production) and social stimulus of strenuous workouts at the gym. There is nothing wrong with this, but strenuous exercise shuts down a fat-burning metabolism. This, of course, is counterproductive to low-carb weight loss efforts since establishing and maintaining a fat-burning metabolism is a key requirement in the LCR.

a) Avoid high-glycemic binging

You know the experience. It's someone's birthday and there is triple death by chocolate, quadruple fudge cake and Haagen-Dazs ice-cream. One serving of this can be hundreds of grams of carbs. Certainly enough to shut down a fat-burning metabolism and create the need to re-establish the keto-lipolytic (fat-burning) process.

Such high-glycemic binging essentially forces the low-carb "dieter" to go through a recovery mode to regain the low-carb weight-loss "ground" that was so hard won. How long this takes and how much effort is uniquely dependent on each person's metabolic makeup and diligence in the recovery process. Although metabolisms and their recovery rates vary, it seems likely, nonetheless, that it may take anywhere from a few days to a week in order to recover from high-glycemic binging.

b) A quick "help" for carb overloading

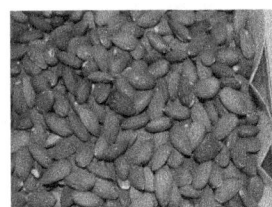 If you make the mistake of blasting your metabolism with high carb food, be sure to also consume protein. As noted before, the Emerald Dry Roasted Almonds are excellent when we need a quick "dose" of delicious protein. They are, also, quite filling.

Do NOT think, however, that you can eat high carb foods followed by some protein and then all will be well: High carb foods MUST be avoided.

However, if you fail, at least give your metabolism some decent protein in order to help ameliorate the blood-sugar spike that will accompany your ingestion of high carb foods.

c) Intentionally going hungry

Another counterproductive "gas and brakes" approach by wayward low-carbers is seeking to lose weight by going hungry. This – of course – activates a body metabolism "starvation" mode which actually shuts down a fat-burning metabolism.

In fairness, the motivation behind going hungry in an effort to lose weight is often quite noble. After all, the common view is "no pain, no gain." For many in this, it is as if they cannot accept losing weight without suffering.

6. A Scene from Sister Act:

This reminds me of the scene from the movie Sister Act in which Sister Mary Clarence (Whoopi Goldberg) commiserates with Sister Mary Lazarus regarding the status of the choir:

Sister Mary Clarence: Mary Lazarus, as soon as I walked through that door I knew that you knew that. Let me ask you something, you're someone in favor of hard work and discipline, right?

Sister Mary Lazarus: Of course, I'm a nun! Four popes now.

Sister Mary Clarence: Four? Wow. Let me ask you, how often do they rehearse?

Sister Mary Lazarus: Twice a week, couple hours.

Sister Mary Clarence: Not enough. I mean listen to them, they really need a lot of work.

Sister Mary Lazarus: Do you really think they could get better?

Sister Mary Clarence: I don't know, they're pretty raw.

Sister Mary Lazarus: Wet behind the ears.

Sister Mary Patrick: Oh please let us try.

Sister Mary Clarence: This is gonna be hell.

Sister Mary Lazarus: Tell me about it.

7. Weight-loss Achievement without GREAT effort:

The exchange is charmingly funny in the film, but my point is that some of us will NOT accept achievement without GREAT effort. The idea of not being hungry, of not exercising strenuously, of getting to eat fat-rich foods instead of the fat-free "cardboard" that passes for "diet" food (the flavour of food is in the fat) just flies in the face of reason for people like Sister Mary Lazarus.

8. Low-Carb without High Healthful Fat & High Protein:

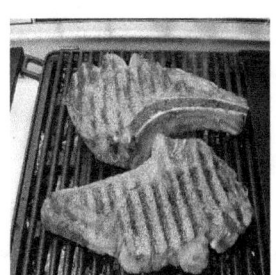 Many are also convinced that eating fat and anything more than modest protein intake is counter to good health (for instance, detrimental to

139

heart health according to conventional wisdom).

Insufficient fat and protein intake thwart a fat-burning metabolism. More to the point, those actually adopting a properly undertaken low-carb regimen tend to report improved blood pressure levels, glucose levels and insulin levels.

Keep in mind that the reasons for adopting the LCR include managing insulin resistance. Weight loss is actually a natural by-product of using the Low-Carb Regimen to deal with this pre-diabetic condition.

9. High carb, High Glycemic Binging:

In addition, most attempting the LCR begin from a "position" of already being addicted to high carb, high glycemic foods.

Many, therefore, seek to reduce some carbs but fail to:

- deal with carb addiction
- adequately increase dietary fat and protein
- eat frequently enough to keep from being hungry, and
- eliminate strenuous exercise (while adding light aerobic exercise)

10. My Testimonial:

Having explained the concepts above, a summary of my personal experience follows:

a) No Dieting!

I never dieted (I can't stand being hungry) I just changed what I ate (mostly got rid of high carb, high glycemic foods and increased proteins, fats, berries, melons, leafy green vegetables, other non-starchy vegetables, and other low-carb/low glycemic foods. I learned to make low-carb pumpkin pie which I eat with homemade whipping cream (made without sugar), low-carb cheesecakes, low-carb breads and muffins, and numerous spectacularly delicious low-carb meals.

b) Bacon!

I learned that fat is my friend when I eat low-carb. Yay: Butter and bacon and cheese!

c) Light Exercise!

I only allowed myself light aerobic exercise and made sure I ate every two hours (I did NOT diet – I feasted up to eight times per day).

d) Rates of Weight-Loss

The obese pounds of the BMI index went really quickly. The top half of the BMI overweight pounds went more slowly while the bottom half of the BMI overweight pounds disappeared most slowly of all (about a half pound or so per week).

If the LCR as detailed in this book is adhered to, the pounds tend to just come off.

The key is getting the body to shift from a carb/sugar energy cycle to a fat burning cycle.

e) Things That Work Against a Fat-Burning Metabolism

Strenuous and/or heavy exercise shuts down the fat burning cycle as does eating high carb, high glycemic foods.

Not eating every few hours also shuts down the fat burning energy cycle.

It is counter-intuitive, but one must eat (in the Low-Carb Regimen) in order to lose weight.

f) Food Flavours!

An interesting plus to the LCR is that – while carb withdrawal only lasts one to three days – the improved flavours of foods may continue. Energy levels may increase and the sense of well-being may elevate: It is remarkable!

III. A Commentary on the Low-Carb Process:

Where will we go from here?

1. What a delight (I achieved my goal during the Christmas season)!

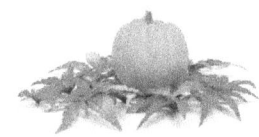

Of course, the absolute best part of the holidays is being with family and friends. Even beyond this, let us always remember the ultimate gift from the One who is the reason for the season!

The gift of life is surprising and astonishing. It is even more so when life is infused with health and vitality.

Consequently, even our gift exchanging was influenced by the low-carb regimen this year. For instance, my wife and I opened our presents to one another while we were having our coffee Christmas morning. I received the gift I desired – a digital scale.

Of course, I had to try it out.

2. Goal reached!

In January 2012, I weighed in at 244 pounds. Christmas morning 2012, I weighed in at 180 (actually at least a pound less since I did not have the benefit of the modest reduction from my weight measuring protocol as described in my Having Fun Stepping on the Scale. To emphasize my point, the morning after Christmas - even though I ate a sumptuous feast for Christmas dinner the night before - I followed my protocol and weighed in at 178 pounds.

As a side note: A week after Christmas and I continue to weigh (as expected) between 178 and 180 pounds.

I appear to have stabilized my weight at this level and continue to enjoy a robust and fulfilling menu of low-carb meals up to eight times per day.

3. The LCR versus "traditional" weight loss:

Frankly, I'm blown away by the results of the Low-Carb Regimen LCR). By comparison, processes used to lose weight in the past either did not work or required arduous discipline that ultimately collapsed under the weight of their demand for unrelenting adherence.

To elaborate, in the past losing weight was a difficult and unpleasant experience with frequent pangs of hunger. You know what I mean: The traditional "dieting" by "starving yourself to lose weight" approach. In the LCR, however, we do not go hungry and instead need to "feed" our ketosis (fat burning) metabolism. In this way I do not diet but instead feast!

Counter-intuitive though it may be, it is necessary to regularly and consistently eat low-carb, high healthful fat, high protein foods in order to succeed in the low-carb regimen.

4. Removing the "hunger barrier" by changing what you eat:

Let me emphasize: The LCR removes the "hunger barrier" to weight loss.

The reason it worked for me was simply a change from destructive food consumption to a very enjoyable, fulfilling and satisfying LCR.

It was really a no-brainer: Get rid of foods that ruin my health, my mental acuity and my energy level. Replace those high glycemic, high carb foods with low glycemic, low-carb, high healthful fat, high protein real foods.

5. Overcoming insulin resistance and discovering flavour:

As I made the change to the LCR everything tasted better (when you stop flooding your taste buds with sugary carbs, the real flavour of healthful foods – previously masked by the carbs – becomes delightfully apparent). In addition, my blood sugar and cholesterol levels optimized (no effort on my part – just a result of healthful low-carb eating).

My pre-diabetic, insulin resistant propensity now is eliminated and controlled by healthful eating.

My energy levels increased. Mental acuity and alertness appear enhanced. The 46 inch "relaxed waist" slacks I used to wear seem laughable compared to the 34 inch "slim fit" Dockers (33 inch in regular cut clothes) that now fit with room to spare. It's a delight to shop for and comfortably wear clothes again!

More to the point, my LCR is so delicious and enjoyable that the high glycemic, sugary carb foods I ate a year ago now have zero appeal. Frankly, I think if I ate them I would feel ill.

6. A beautiful secret:

This introduces a beautiful secret: Once we have actually adapted to healthful low-carb eating we won't want to go back to eating the addictive junk that makes us overweight. This is the real bonus to Step Five of our LCR:

7. Adding back low glycemic, relatively low-carb foods:

Now that I've reached Step Five of my LCR I'm having tons of fun adding back low glycemic, relatively low-carb foods.

Here's an example of my application of maintaining (once we have reached our weight loss goal) in the low-carb eating regimen. My Christmas dinner included (all of these are relatively low-carb and homemade):

- Rum and maple flavored butter and Stevia glazed baked ham.

- Fresh pineapple and cranberry butter fried sweet potatoes with Vietnamese cinnamon.

Note: Sweet potatoes and pineapple are NOT low-carb foods. However, they are healthful and may be eaten occasionally if eaten in moderation.

- Sautéed onion and bacon fried green beans.

- Broccoli cooked in my world class cheese sauce.

- Fresh cranberry and navel orange relish.

- Homemade date and coconut flour biscuits topped with real cream butter.

- Dill pickle spears.

- Unsweetened, unflavored coconut milk lattes.

- Hot ginger steeped tea.

- Homemade New York style low-carb cheesecake.

- Almond flour-crusted, low-carb pumpkin pie with whipped cream.

Wow, what a feast!

Chapter Eight Conclusion – Time to eat and to work out:

As described in this chapter, Step Five - Maintaining means getting to continue in the delightful process of the LCR. Once we have achieved the BMI ideal weight that applies to us as individuals, we stop eating to lose weight and instead eat to maintain the benefits of relatively low-carb nutrition. It is important, however, to remind oneself periodically of the principles that create those benefits.

After all, we live in a carb-addicted society and we need to guard against sliding back into high-glycemic patterns.

As noted before, another delight in the Low-Carb Regimen is that we eat every few hours (up to eight times per day).

It's been a few hours. Time for another latte and some of my delicious low-carb pumpkin pie topped with whipped cream!

But first I think I'll do a light aerobic workout!

Chapter Nine

Does A Low-Carb Diet Really Work?

As Answered By The "My Big Fat Diet" Research

The chapter you are reading – by far the briefest in this book – is the "video" section of the Low-Carb Regimen. In this chapter we focus on a recent documentary that establishes the effectiveness of a low-carb diet in general. Even though the low-carb diet of the documentary differs in a number of ways from our Low-Carb Regimen (LCR), the videos validate a large scale, low-carb approach to weight-loss.

I. My Big Fat Diet

If you are concerned about weight loss, diabetes, heart disease, cancer or if you simply would like to adopt an eating regimen that may have success against these enemies of health, then you will absolutely want to see the "My Big Fat Diet" video (the links are included two paragraphs below).

Per the About.com, Low-Carb Diets article, **My Big Fat Diet** is a fascinating documentary of the work performed by Métis physician, **Dr. Jay Wortman**, with the cooperation of nearly one hundred participants from the Namgis first nation in Alert Bay, British Columbia,

Canada. Dr. Wortman sought to return the participants to a more traditional diet by seeking to eliminate the sugars and carbohydrates introduced by Europeans and increasingly adopted into the cultural diet of first nation members.

Those interested in viewing the documentary will be pleased to discover that the My Big Fat Diet video, Parts –

- **One** (http://www.youtube.com/watch?v=bjTmdvFH3gQ),

- **Two** (http://www.youtube.com/watch?v=RZy8atek8dg)

- **Three** (http://www.youtube.com/watch?v=6Bnw-TjpkaI)

– is available through YouTube per the provided links.

Dr. Wortman's research would surely have been applauded by **Dr. Weston Price** who introduced the concept of the "ancestral" diet in his landmark 1939 book **Nutrition and Physical Degeneration** and **Dr. Robert Atkins** who is – of course – the originator of the famed **Atkins diet**.

Chapter Ten

Food Supplements That Support

A Low-Carb Regimen (LCR) Lifestyle

Adequate nourishment is a key concern for any diet. To ensure sufficient nutrition in our low-carb lifestyle, the following discussion and review of food supplements is offered:

I. Just Give Me A Pill

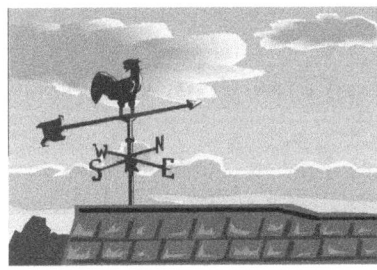

One of the difficulties with foods available for consumption is finding foods with truly adequate nutritional compositions. Simply put, our foods may look good, but they may not be "as good as they look" from a nutritional standpoint.

In consideration of this, some seek to augment their nutritional intake with food supplements. Food supplements have grown to a multi-billion dollar industry.

Those opposed to this trend protest that food supplements at best create expensive urine. To this a nutritionist I once knew replied, "Expensive urine is what we want!" (If the subtle point presented in the preceding exchange isn't registering, the idea is that it is a good thing to have such a rich nutritional surplus in your diet that your body can afford to shed nutrients!)

More in sync with contemporary society is the idea that we want everything to be fixed by just taking a pill. From my perspective, this is part of the "fad" stampede as exemplified by individuals rushing to purchase raspberry ketone supplements when Dr. Oz promoted them on his television show.

Although food supplements are merely classified as foods, even so, individuals taking them should be careful to follow the guidelines given by the manufacturers and distributors of those products. With this in mind, I do take food supplements as needed. Some that I have found effective are listed below:

1. Per Chapter Six: Did You Ger Your Vitamin D?

The link is to Spring Valley Vitamin D-3 softgels.

As noted in Chapters One and Six, elimination of milk also eliminates the Vitamin D supplementation that is added to milk by the Dairy Industry. For emphasis, **insufficient daily Vitamin D** can interfere with healthful metabolism and low-carb weight loss.

2. Calcium Pantothenate (aka: Pantothenic Acid)

The link is to TwinLab's version of Vitamin B-5 as marketed through Walgreens. This supplement appears to stimulate the oxygen transport capacity of hemoglobin to the brain and in this way promotes alertness. For many this supplement works like a strong cup of coffee (without the caffeine side-affects). However, the body does appear to adapt to the use of this supplement (and then it's just a good source of certain nutrients). As a result, ongoing supplementation is unlikely to continue to produce the same "alertness" result. Therefore, using this supplement on occasion, or even for a few days, may be beneficial. Subsequent discontinuance for a few days is suggested before resumption of B-5 supplementation.

It would seem logical that individuals suffering from high blood pressure would want to exercise caution in taking supplements that could impact blood transport. As with all things related to health, consultation with a doctor may be advised.

Again, the "big wow" for calcium pantothenate is its ability to promote alertness when we are fatigued. I can testify that when I am fighting through a mental fog, this supplement seems to really help!

3. Garlic Oil Capsules

Garlic oil capsules are believed to stimulate the immune system. Maximum effect appears to result from the capsules containing the actual garlic oil rather than from tablets. Walmart markets twin packs of two bottles of 1000 mg softgels from the Spring Valley company for a mere $6.00 (way to go, Walmart!). I take two capsules of garlic oil daily for immune support.

When I was ill as a youngster, my grandparents would give me raw garlic for the same purpose touted for these supplements. Trust me: The softgels are so much more pleasant to take AND the softgels per the link above are "odorless."

Capsules that are not odorless may produce olfactory insults for those who must be around you!

4. Echinacea Capsules

Echinacea capsules are also touted for immune system support. Walmart's Spring Valley product provides 250 capsules at a cost of $9.00. The marketing information for this product claims:

The Spring Valley Natural Echinacea Supplement is a blend of different combinations of essential natural vitamins, minerals and plant extracts. This herbal supplement is the most effective and convenient way to provide consistent amounts of specific nutrients and helps reach the level of optimal health. This immune health supplement are used for treating various health disorders like high blood pressure, boosting energy, preventing diseases and regulating vital body functions. This Echinacea supplement, a primary herb used to cleanse and detox your lymphatic system.

5. CoQ10 200 mg Capsules

My link for this supplement is from NatureMade. Among other things, the supplement appears to stimulate energy levels. At nearly twenty dollars for a bottle of 40 softgels, this is – for me – a more expensive supplement, but I believe the benefit outweighs the cost.

According to **Livestrong.com**:

CoQ10 is everywhere

Coenzyme C10, or CoQ10, is present in every cell in plants and animals. It helps improve energy function and acts as an antioxidant, interrupting the damage of free radicals. It can help prevent cancer and heart disease in healthy people and has a number of uses in different diseases. CoQ10 levels are twice as high in vegetarians as in omnivores because it is present in high levels in plant foods. Most studies of CoQ10 have used a dosage of 100 mg per day, but doctors use doses up to 300 mg per day in patients with severe heart disease. A good rule of thumb is to take 2 mg for each kilogram (2.2 lbs.) of body weight.

In addition the article claims that:

- CoQ10 promotes heart health
- CoQ10 aids in the control of diabetes
- CoQ10 aids in the prevention of gum disease

- CoQ10 aids in cancer care

6. Activated Charcoal Capsules

My link is to the Nature's Way activated charcoal capsules that market through Walgreens. Each bottle contains one hundred 280 mg softgels. These are amazingly useful for upset stomachs. Activated charcoal capsules are hands down the best product I have ever used for this purpose.

Note: The instructions with the activated charcoal supplement clearly indicate that it will absorb minerals and possibly other nutrients as well. Consequently, charcoal supplements may also interfere with the absorption of any medicines that you may take. Most who use this supplement use it sparingly and not for extended time periods.

You might find it interesting to note that in the days of westward expansion by American settlers (in the 1800s) savvy pioneer moms would burn a piece of toast when a youngster had an upset stomach. This created a "natural" activated charcoal which in turn produced a similar effect to the activated charcoal capsules referenced above. I can testify that the capsules are better than the burnt toast!

In a more extreme circumstance, many Emergency Rooms keep powdered activated charcoal available for poisoning cases.

7. Raspberry Ketone Capsules

As noted above, **raspberry ketone capsules** were highlighted by the Dr. Oz show last April. His website states: "Metabolic-boosting raspberry ketone is a compound found in red raspberries; it basically slices up fat cells, making them easier to be burned as fuel. These ketones also help keep you feeling full and help to keep cravings under control. Raspberry ketones are better taken as a supplement because you would need to eat 1000 raspberries to reap the same benefits. Aim for 100 mg before lunch and again at dinner. Look for raspberry ketones layered in a supplement with other fat-fighting ingredients."

Caution: Price gouging in supplement sales is common. I've seen raspberry ketone supplements typically offered at ten to twenty dollars per bottle. I also know of at least one site that charges nearly sixty dollars per bottle (for essentially the same product as the others). I encourage buyers to beware when it comes to purchasing all things including food supplements!

8. Zinc Tablets

I was introduced to this supplement because of its support for the body's healing process and because it is often deficient in men. If you look at your fingernails and see small patches of "white clouds" under the nails, you may be deficient in zinc. It should also be noted that zinc supplementation may stimulate sex drive.

9. Magnesium Tablets

If you find that your thoughts seem to churn in disarray and that you have difficulty concentrating, you might benefit from magnesium supplements. I have found them to be useful for support with pain management and for concentration filtering.

10. Vitamin C

Most of us do not get sufficient vitamin C. Vitamin C may be effective in fluid transport. It has been described by some as a "vacuum cleaner" that aids in disposing of waste materials through the urine.

11. Probiotics

The healthy bacteria in our gut is a foundational line of defense against illness. Regular consumption of foods – such as yogurt – containing probiotics is a good start, but many supplement this process by purchasing and using **probiotic softgels**.

12. Calcium

If we consume a couple of glasses daily of **So Delicious unsweetened, unflavoured coconut milk**, we will support our calcium needs. We also have good sources of calcium through the many delicious cheeses and butter that we consume.

Presuming, then, that we have obtained decent quality food supplements, do they really work?

Burt Wolf comments in one of his travel videos on the perceived impact of drinking hot chocolate. Some cultures believe hot chocolate will help you relax while others think it will help you become more alert. Amazingly, the perception of those drinking the beverage tends to match their cultural expectations.

One should not discount the psychosomatic influence of one's actions, nor should one discount the well-documented placebo effect. Having observed these things – based on experience and research that I have read – I believe the supplements listed above impact me in the ways described.

Chapter Eleven
"So, Where's My Bread?"
Low-Carb Flours in the Fight for "the Battle of the Bulge"

You won't get too far into your quest to follow a low-carb eating regimen before you wonder, "Where's my bread?"

The answer is you can buy it (expensive, rarely fresh and sometimes hard to find) or you can make it (depending on the result you'll accept, this can be difficult).

Note: Baking your own low-carb breads, biscuits and pancakes is much simpler with the recent development and more accessible marketing of true low-carb flour. See the **Carbquik Bake Mix** high fiber flour at **netrition.com**.

Also, please note that **Step Five** – Maintaining A Low-Carb Regimen For A Lifetime is for those who have achieved their Low-Carb Regimen (LCR) weight-loss goal and who are now seeking to maintain their weight. It is possible that true low-carb flours may stimulate "carb craving," a result that is counterproductive to the first four steps of the Low-Carb Regimen (LCR).

I. Making your own low-carb breads

1. Making your own low-carb breads can be challenging

The reason is that all traditional baking flours are loaded with carbs!

2. If you truly want to eat low-carb

– and if you rule out soy and glutens (my wife is allergic to these) – you are essentially left with "meals" made from nuts (almond meal, coconut meal, flaxseed meal and hazelnut meal). To this you can add oat fiber though oat fiber is actually a dietary supplement intended to increase fiber intake.

a) These "meals" (sometimes called "flours") in and of themselves can be pricey

I've seen almond meal flour for ten to fifteen dollars per pound, though it can be purchased locally at Whole Foods in their bulk container aisle for about five dollars per pound.

b) Since you are no longer cooking with gluten, breads will tend to crumble

School house glue was originally a white flour paste (made sticky because of the gluten in the flour). As a result, breads without gluten do tend to crumble. One way to overcome this is to increase the number of eggs in the recipe. A caution here, however: Too many eggs can create a quiche!

3. In the Low-Carb Cooking Guide at the end of this book

I've included the recipe for a **low-carb loaf** (more like a banana bread loaf without the bananas because they are loaded with carbs, too). Keep in mind this "bread" is NOT at all like the commercially available sandwich breads that one buys from your local grocery store. On the other hand, it can be used very much like those commercially available, high carb breads.

4. Having said these things, what is the math on the net carb counts of various flours and meals?

Consider the following two tables:

Type of flour or meal	Serving Size	Total Carbs	Fiber	Net Carbs
almond	1/4 cup	6	3	3
amaranth	1/4 cup	20	3	17
barley	1/4 cup	23	5	18
buckwheat	1/4 cup	21	4	17
coconut	1/4 cup	16	10	6
flaxseed meal	1/4 cup	4	4	0
hazlenut meal	1/4 cup	5	3	2
kamut	1/4 cup	21	3	18
millet	1/4 cup	22	4	18
oat	1/4 cup	26	4	22
oat fiber	100 grams	91	90	1

Type of flour or meal	Serving Size	Total Carbs	Fiber	Net Carbs
potato	1/4 cup	36	3	33
rice	1/4 cup	31	2	29
rye	1/4 cup	21	1	20
quinoa	1/4 cup	18	2	16
seminola	1/4 cup	30	1	29
sorghum	1/4 cup	25	3	22
soy	1/4 cup	8	3	5
spelt	1/4 cup	22	4	18
tapioca	1/4 cup	26	0	26
tricale	1/4 cup	23	5	18
unbleached white	1/4 cup	21	1	20
whole wheat	1/4 cup	23	4	19

From the tables it is easy to see why traditional flours are avoided in a low-carb regimen!

II. Buying low-carb breads

1. Another low-carb perspective answer to the question, "So, where's my bread?"

Low-carb breads are available if you know where to get them, if cost is not a problem, and if you do not require homemade. Again, keep in mind that many of these low-carb breads contain soy, gluten or both.

2. Here is where you can find some of the pre-made, low-carb breads:

Wholefoods and Sprouts Farmer's Markets are good local (Colorado Springs) options. Online via Amazon is another.

a) Julian Bakery **markets online a popular, 1 net carb per slice bread:**

http://www.julianbakery.com/lc-promo/

b) Health Express markets (online via Amazon) several low-carb breads ranging from eight to ten dollars per loaf.

These include:

Health Express All Natural 3 Net Carb **Cinnamon Almond Raisin Bread**(2 Loaves)

Health Express All Natural 1 Net Carb **Flax Seed Bread** (Pack of 3 Loaves)

Health Express 1 Net Carb **All Natural Bread**

Health Express All Natural 1 Net Carb **Oat Bran Bread** (Pack of 3 Loaves)

Carb Krunchers also markets online via Amazon a low-carb bread:

Carb Krunchers Low-Carb **Everything Bread (Pack of 2)**

3. Additional products made by these companies include breadsticks, rolls, and biscuits.

If you are not set on homemade and your budget allows, I encourage you to explore these products.

Finally, keep in mind that the Low-Carb Regimen – among other things – is a long term process in which the insulin resistant seek to facilitate the body's ability to reduce accumulated fat by the appropriate reduction of carbs in the diet.

In many ways this is a "battle of the bulge" and – as noted – the question of "where is the bread" in this process, though a challenge, is at least manageable!

III. Yeast Bread for the Low-Carb Regimen

In the process of avoiding carbohydrates we find ourselves cutting back – or eliminating altogether – the breads that are so much a part of contemporary diets.

Sadly, there are not many alternatives that are bread AND are low-carb. However, there is a **low-carb yeast bread** in the **1 To 5 Low-Carb Cooking Guide**!

Flatbread Variations

If you are alright with flatbread, check out Mission's **Carb Balance Whole Wheat Small Fajita Tortillas**.

Traditionally these are used for fajitas, tacos, enchiladas, burritos, and quesadillas.

In addition, use them for sandwich rollups, rolled up by themselves, or stacked on top of each other to make more conventional (though, round) sandwiches. If you are determined to have a still more conventional shape, the stacked tortillas – into which you have placed your favourite sandwich ingredients – can be readily trimmed into a rectangular form that more closely resembles a conventional sandwich.

Another variation is to spread a filling on the tortilla, roll the tortilla up, and then cut the tortilla into a series of pinwheels.

A more ambitious option is to make your own low-carb "bread."

As noted before, the "breads" that I make are really more "loaves" similar to a banana bread loaf.

The reason for this is that while wheat flours work well with yeast, virtually all flours – especially wheat flours – are loaded with carbs. An exception is almond flour (though technically almond flour is actually a "meal" made from ground almonds). Oat flour is relatively low in carbohydrates compared to other flours. Vital wheat gluten is lower in net carbs than typical wheat flours and can be used in small quantities (depending on your daily net carb needs and your ability to tolerate gluten) to bake bread.

The benefit of using some form of wheat in your homemade bread is that your leavening (your yeast) functions correctly in wheat flours. It can be extremely difficult to get meals and non-wheat whole grains to rise through the action of yeast.

Milled flax seed has zero net carbs and is a decent source of protein. I like to add some milled flax seed as a "coating" to the outside of my raised bread dough. It adds protein, fiber and a nice, rustic texture. Sesame seeds are good for this purpose as well.

Now that we've considered the matter of our daily bread, let's look at some great Low-Carb Regimen beverages. Hydration is extremely important in the Low-Carb Regimen but – obviously – not all beverages are low-carb.

Chapter Twelve
Drink One For Yourself:
A Few Beverages To Drink Right Now

I am the proud owner of a Dutch Brothers "Drink One for Dane" t-shirt.

Dutch Brothers? The Low-Carb Regimen? "Drink one for Dane," you ask?

Here's the story:

Each year Dutch Brothers Coffee locations host MDA Day, donating all proceeds to the Muscular Dystrophy Association (MDA), a nonprofit organization dedicated to curing muscular dystrophy, ALS and related diseases by funding worldwide research.

The event, which kicked off ALS Awareness Month, is held annually in honor of company co-founder, Dane Boersma, who was diagnosed with ALS in 2005 and passed away in late 2009.

Additionally, Dutch Brothers gave away MDA stickers. (Mine is proudly displayed on the right rear of my car!) Customers were also able to make donations at danesdrive.org.

So why all the fuss about Dutch Brothers when this book is about the Low-Carb Regimen (LCR)?

I. A Few Beverages to Drink RIGHT Now

1. Coffee:

Coffee has received some nice "pats on the back" from researchers. Since my family has a Dutch / Swedish connection, this created an interest in Dutch Brothers coffee.

More to the point, the good news for java drinkers is that coffee has virtually no carbohydrates.

This is NOT true of milk:

Milk from skim to whole is loaded with carbs . . .

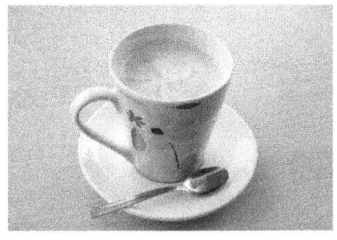

From a low-carb eating perspective this means that you can have a cup of coffee and it does not increase your carb load so long as you eliminate the milk and the sweeteners.

Cream is not quite so bad (remember, fat is our friend and cream tends to be added to coffee in small amounts), but if you really want to be carb conscious, eliminate the cream, too, and either drink your coffee black, or:

Use unsweetened almond milk or unsweetened coconut milk.

In a pinch, if you need a sweetener in your coffee you could use some Stevia. Keep in mind, however, that there is a train of thought within the low-carb eating movement that all sweeteners (including the artificial ones) behave in the body like carbs.

Therefore, moderation is encouraged.

2. Hot Tea:

I became a tea drinker as a youngster (I grew up in a British Commonwealth country – my parents' fault!).

Tea is also virtually carb free, and – if you need to eliminate the caffeine – herbal teas can be excellent.

West a ways from Denver is the college community of Boulder. There you can make arrangements to tour the Celestial Seasonings home base. It is worth the tour, and the teas are good, too!

3. Iced Tea:

Arizona Tea markets a Diet (decaffeinated, if you prefer) Green Tea sweetened with Splenda that I personally like. But – if artificial sweeteners behave in the body like sugar (the grand daddy of all carbohydrates), then it is good to avoid artificially sweetened teas. I have found, however, that "cutting" the tea with water (I use a ratio of about one fifth tea to four fifths water) and then adding a slice of either fresh lime or fresh lemon (do NOT use lemon or lime juice – too high in carbohydrates!) makes a wonderful, refreshing, flavourful beverage.

You can also easily brew your own teas or herbal teas and create very healthful and flavourful iced or hot teas!

4. AVOID hot or cold "store bought" chocolate beverages:

They tend to be loaded with carbs! Baking cocoa, on the other hand, is relatively low in carbs. It is what we do with the original cocoa in order to make it appealing to our tastes that loads chocolate beverages and confections with carbohydrates.

5. Unsweetened, unflavoured coconut or almond milk:

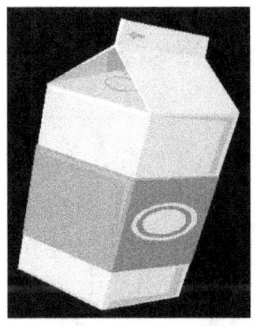 I really like the **unsweetened, unflavoured coconut milk**: Not only is it nearly carb free (there is only 1 net carb in an eight ounce glass!), but – to me – it tastes great when I make my latte.

I also like a cold glass of unsweetened coconut milk straight up.

My wife likes the unsweetened, vanilla flavoured almond milk which she then sweetens with Stevia. She regularly has a glass with dinner and finds it delicious! As noted before, I have found the almond milk imparts an unpleasant "wheat-like" flavour to lattes.

I can't really speak about soy milk (my wife is allergic to soy, so we never use it).

Rice milk is made from a starchy carbohydrate and we seek to avoid these.

6. The Right Milk for Lattes:

Not all brands and varieties of unsweetened coconut milk taste the same in a latte.

I like the **So Delicious brand unsweetened, unflavoured coconut milk** in lattes. On the other hand, I find the vanilla flavoured and sweetened (not great for carbs anyway) creates a miserable flavour with coffee. Of course, suit yourself in this regard but, again, the coconut milk that I like in my latte is the unsweetened, unflavoured coconut milk.

7. Water:

Allowing for filtration of hazardous materials from your water, a good, cold glass of water is the gold standard for thirst.

It should be noted that – in the history of soft beverages (hard ones evidently always have been a hit with those who wanted to "loosen up") – it was originally difficult to get people to buy soft drinks. Coca Cola was the first (it was popularly believed that Coca Cola originally was made lawfully with small quantities of what are now illicit drugs). In any case, it was a tough sell to get people to pay for soft drinks because one could drink water for free and consumers had not yet become addicted to the taste and the image of soft beverages.

Times have changed, marketing has programmed our brains, and now people will rarely drink just water, preferring instead almost any flavoured beverage or "specialty" water.

(If the event was set in modern times, do you think Adam and Eve would have a soft drink along with the fruit from the tree of the knowledge of good and evil? Not only was eating that fruit – the kind of fruit is never specifically stated – a forbidden act, but if the fruit was an apple, it was high carb!)

8. AVOID soft drinks:

I used to play tennis with a retired MD who (although I am much younger than the retired doctor) regularly ran me off the court. At that time I was putting away a pack of diet coke a day. The retired doctor told me: If you want to lose weight, stop drinking soda pop – especially diet sodas. I believe the good doctor was right and the Low-Carb Regimen supports this idea!

9. Lemon or lime infused water:

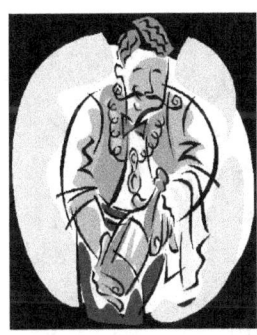 There's an important trick here: The squeezed juice from a lemon or a lime is relatively high in carbs. You can achieve a lower carb impact (and still get the lemon or lime flavour) by putting a few slices of the lemon or lime (or both) into a pitcher of water and letting it sit in the refrigerator.

Note: Infused water is NOT water with juice added to it; instead, infused water is water in which slices of the whole fruit are allowed to sit and permeate the liquid.

Be sure to clean the lemon, lime or strawberry fruit thoroughly before slicing it into your water for infusion purposes: Keep in mind the dangers from the excess quantities of pesticides, "growth promoting" chemicals and other "undesirables" that are a part of the American food processing chain!

10. Strawberry infused water:

Strawberries – by sliced volume – are relatively (for a fruit) low in carbs.

Clean a few strawberries, slice them into a pitcher, and let the strawberry infused water chill in your refrigerator. Then enjoy – delicious!

11. Juices tend to be high in carbohydrates:

Since juices are the concentrated portions of the "sugary" component of the food, most juices are high in carbohydrates. Therefore, juices should be avoided or – at the very least – minimized.

As an interesting aside in this debate, Dr. Weston Price, a globetrotting dentist keenly involved in the nutritional struggles of a bygone age argued against "partitioning" foods. Partitioned foods are not "whole." In other words, instead of consuming the whole food, we eat only a concentrated (partitioned) portion of the whole food. The argument ran that, "you wouldn't eat eight oranges in one sitting, so why consume the juice of eight oranges?"

An important aside: Oranges, apples, bananas and most fruits are loaded with carbs. From a Low-Carb Eating Regimen perspective strawberries, raspberries, cranberries and blueberries are better choices when eaten in moderation.

If Dr. Price makes a valid argument, then that argument supports the idea that juices are a problem for the insulin resistant.

Regardless of the validity of Dr. Price's observations regarding partitioned foods, from a Low-Carb Eating Regimen perspective the concentrated carbohydrates are to be avoided (or again, at least, minimized).

II. A Few Closing Thoughts

1. Be CAREFUl with carbs and servings in protein "shakes":

Most protein powders and ready made protein shakes are loaded with carbs. A serving may also be just a part of a ready-to-drink "shake" container and – if you drink the entire beverage (as most do) – you load yourself with carbs.

As a result most of these "fitness" drinks (from a Low-Carb Eating Regimen perspective) promote fat production for the insulin resistant. This is obviously the opposite result that most people seek.

On the other hand, the Atkins Advantage Vanilla Shake truly is low-carb (1 gram of net carbs). I like to take some with me when I mountain bike the North Santa Fe trail. It's also a convenient meal replacement when teaching duties eliminate my lunch.

2. Keep yourself hydrated:

In all of this keep in mind that hydration is important on many fronts including electrolyte balance: Make sure you intake sufficient fluids each day, and – while you're at it – drink flavourful, nutritious, delicious, low-carb beverages.

Finally, as in the beginning of this chapter, if you are willing "to drink one for Dane," remember, also, to drink healthfully for yourself!

Chapter Thirteen
A Few Things To Eat Right Now

An eastern parable reminds us that a man who waits to dig a well until he is thirsty will die of thirst!

I would argue that maintaining a healthy, low-carb diet can be like that parable. We need convenient, quick and easy, accessible and acceptable foods that we can eat at the drop of a hat.

Here are a few that I have found helpful:

I. Pre-packaged Foods

Pre-cooked, microwavable bacon and a nice slice of Cheddar cheese give a flavourful, filling and quick input of protein and fat. Some like the convenience of string cheese.

Others prefer a whey shake (Read the label and be sure your whey is low carb!).

I like to make mine with vanilla flavoured whey. Unsweetened, unflavoured coconut milk sliced with really cold water mix well with the whey powder. Pumpkin pie spice makes a great flavouring. Top it off with a dusting of nutmeg!

In addition, the following pre-packaged foods are quick and easy:

1. Number one on my list of "ready when I am" foods is:

Emerald **100 Calorie Packs Dry Roasted Almonds**:

These are available at Walmart though you might have to search a bit or ask for help. Keep in mind that the dry roasted Emerald's version is lowest carb. Each box contains seven packages and the nuts are VERY chewy. I suggest eating them one or two almonds at a time until done. Then give yourself a few moments and you will feel full. The net carb count is only two grams per packet, so – if you are ravenously hungry – you can indulge in a second packet as needed. In addition, at about $3.29 per box (yep, only 47 cents per packet!), you can afford the indulgence!

2. Second on my list is:

No-Sugar **Jello Cups**

With these – of course – you need access to a refrigerator or – in my case – a soft, portable lunch cooler (mine lets me put the long lasting blue ice packs in the lid). The No-Sugar Jello Cups retail in packages of 6 or 12 for about $2.50 and contain zero grams of carbohydrates! I especially like the lime and orange flavoured Jello cups and I made points with my grandson by saving him one of my favourite lime cups for when he came over a few days ago.

3. Third on my list is:

Mission **Carb Balance Small Fajita Whole Wheat Tortillas**

Each tortilla has only 3 grams of net carbs. I find eight-packs of these at Safeway for about $3.84 and so each tortilla is only about 48 cents! The package is a resealable zip lock style bag and – like a loaf of bread – it does not need to be refrigerated. Rolled up, they make a great meal, and – if you've got the condiments – a little butter, almond butter or cream cheese will add some nice variety. I like to keep a bag of these in my desk drawer at work!

4. Fourth on my list is:

Krogger **Carbmaster Yogurt Cups**

I pick these up at our local King Soopers. The flavour selection for these yogurts is diverse and outstanding: They even have carrot cake! Each six ounce cup is only four carbs so you can afford to indulge!

Of course it helps to be prepared for snacks like yogurt and Jello. So make sure you have a spoon available (something else I like to keep in my desk drawer at work!).

Along these lines is the wonderful, old story about a farmland church set in an area that had been going through a drought. The church people decided to hold an outdoor service to pray for the much needed rain but only one little girl actually brought an umbrella . . .

In out case it would seem if we believe we might be hungry, we should bring the needed utensils!

II. Foods I Prepare in Advance

1. Number one on my list of foods I like to make in advance is

Chicken (or any other prepared in advance meat you have on hand)!

As a meat there are essentially no carbs and I can make it in a host of different ways. For instance, I just made another batch of the "Filleted Chicken" per the Low-Carb Cooking Guide located at the end of this book. There are now three portions of this indescribably delicious chicken in separate sealed containers ready to go in my refrigerator. I'm looking forward to the feast!

2. Number two on this list is

Bell Pepper Spears (NOT apple slices: They are loaded with carbs!)

I love to have green, red and orange Bell peppers cut into strips and waiting in my refrigerator in sealed bags: So crunchy, so filling and so flavourful!

3. Number three on my list is

Scintillating Salads!

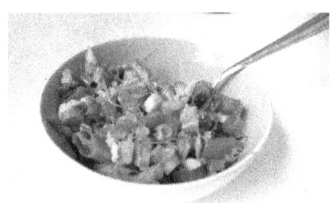

We go nuts on our salads – literally! Along with romaine and spinach we like peppers, broccoli, cucumbers, almonds, sliced strawberries, feta and . . . you get the idea! Just have a portion in an easy storage container that will be ready when you are.

4. Number four on my list is

Any low-carb leftover meal!

If we'll take the time on the weekend to prepare in advance extra portions of meals planned for that week, we will then be ready to rock and roll down the daily aisles of our work week. And – if you know how good it's going to taste (because YOU made it low-carb, nutritious and delicious!) – it can be a lot of fun getting it together!

Again for an excellent meal see the Low-Carb Cooking Guide **split chicken breast recipe** in the back of this book.

Chapter Fourteen
LCR Maintenance, Health Bulletin,
High Glycemic Binging and Anti-Aging

I. The Low-Carb Maintenance – Step Five – Applied:

1. Having Fun Stepping on the Scale

After arising this morning and going through my **"Having Fun Stepping on the Scale"** regimen, my weight continues to maintain at my target of 179 pounds.

So, my "Step Five: Maintaining a LCR for a Lifetime" by continuing to add back low glycemic, healthful, relatively low-carb foods is on track!

2. Denser Muscle Tissue

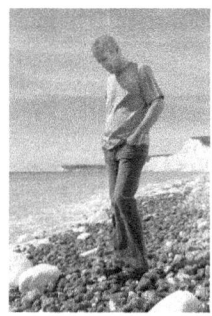 In addition, I have added back more strenuous, muscle building exercises via my **Gold's XRS 30** home gym: What a delight to have the light aerobic conditioning in place that makes my twenty minute Gold's gym regimen a pleasant stressing of my major muscle

groups. It should be noted, however, that heavier exercises convert fat to muscle AND muscle tissue is more dense than fat tissue which in turn adds density (and weight) to your body IF you maintain the same body volume.

3. A Relatively Low-Carb Breakfast

I enjoyed my before and after breakfast unsweetened, unflavoured coconut milk lattes (I grind my espresso beans fresh!). The lattes went well with my low-carb version of the traditional American breakfast of two eggs over easy on top of a homemade **low-carb biscuit** with butter and lots of **sausage and gravy**.

4. A Low-Carb Dinner

Last night I treated myself to my wonderful **low-carb homemade New York style cheesecake**.

For dinner my wife and I feasted on my homemade **New England style clam chowder**. This recipe can be varied to make a soup similar to Olive Garden's Sausage and Kale Soup (**Zoupa Tuscana**).

II. A LCR Health Bulletin

Frequently in the news is the annual flu season and regular onslaughts of the norovirus.

1. Health Bulletin

The norovirus remains a highly contagious threat that seems to just keep making the rounds each year, but attention to this Health Bulletin allows a healthful low-carb response.

Both of these illnesses can impact those who seek the benefits of a LCR. Here's how:

2. Gastro-Intestinal Challenges for LCRs

In the LCR we seek to convert our bodies to fat-burning (keto-genesis) rather than fat-storing metabolisms (carbohydrate-glucose-insulin: CGI).

Fat stores, however, are useful when dealing with illness – particularly illnesses that destroy our appetites and our desire for hydration. Keep in mind that effective low-carb eating requires "feasting" every few hours along with healthy and regular intake of fluids. The norovirus, in particular (but the flu, potentially, as well) can interfere with our regular intake of healthful foods and fluids.

3. Seeing your doctor without delay

The result can be a dramatic drop in fluid levels and energy reserves which in turn can cause a precipitous drop in blood pressure. This can cause loss of balance – in some cases actually passing out with an accompanying fall to the ground along with collateral damage associated with such falls.

As a caution, then, those on a Low-Carb Eating Regimen who find that eating and hydrating every few hours is undesirable as a result of illness will want to find a way to appropriately ingest adequate nourishment and fluid or make it a priority to quickly see their doctor.

4. The BRAT diet and adequate fluids

A classic aid in dealing with gastrointestinal distress is the well-known "BRAT" diet. BRAT, of course is an acronym for "bananas, rice, applesauce and toast." These foods are not low-carb, but when dealing with these diseases: Nourishment and fluids first, low-carb later. Fluids useful for electrolyte support are also suggested. There are Splenda versions of Gatorade and other sport beverages. "Flat" ginger ale (ginger ale that has lost its carbonation) is suggested by some. Water with sliced fruit also may be of use and some commend the Airborne products.

5. Low-carb eating concerns for pregnant or lactating women:

In line with these nutritional concerns when dealing with illness, it should also be observed that pregnant or lactating women – regardless of trending diseases – will want to follow the nutritional guidelines established for their respective conditions rather than embracing a Low-Carb Eating Regimen.

III. High Glycemic Binging

1. Well-Intentioned Low-Carbers

On another "front" I continue to find well-intentioned low-carbers who seek to use the LCR as a means to indulge sporadic, binge carbaholism. You know what I mean: Those who periodically "jump off the low-carb bandwagon" and eat high glycemic "foods" with the attitude that "being really good about low-carb eating" for a period of time makes it alright to abuse their metabolisms with high carb foods.

2. Net-Carb Errors

The fallacy to this approach is much like the error of those who think that adding fiber to foods lowers the net carb count of that food. To review, since fiber is carbohydrate, adding fiber to food (while potentially beneficial in many ways) merely adds an equal amount of carbohydrate and does NOT reduce the net carb count of the food to which the fiber is added.

3. Cyclic Low-Carb Errors

In much the same way cyclically "jumping on" and "jumping off" the LCR "vehicle" makes it extremely difficult to maintain a fat burning metabolism. It is NOT true that you can "make up" for high glycemic binging with "really eating low-carb well" in spurts. A fat burning metabolism is for most a delicately balanced metabolic engine that requires ongoing participation rather than "fits and starts" of on again off again adherence.

4. Truly Overcoming Carb Withdrawal

Those who need cyclic high glycemic binging have not successfully overcome carb withdrawal (either physically, mentally, emotionally or some combination of the three). It is suggested that if you are in this "state" – and if you desire success in the Low-Carb Eating Regimen – you may benefit from going back to Step One of the Low-Carb Eating Regimen and truly mastering overcoming carb withdrawal . . .

5. High Glycemic Errors

Keep in mind that part of overcoming carb withdrawal is getting to the spot where high glycemic foods are seen as the potential "poisons" that they actually are.

See the April 2013 TED **presentation by Dr. Peter Attia** for a converted low-carb MD's take on high glycemic, highly refined carbohydrates. He also introduces "insulin resistance," the topic of **Chapter Fifteen** in this book.

It may help to think of high glycemic foods as being like "hemlock." Would you crave hemlock? Of course not! Or, if you did, then your mental health would be seriously suspect!

And herein lies the difficulty of our culture and the images that advertising have imprinted into our thinking: It is so easy to desire that which is destructive (because our culture and advertising make destructive things look VERY appealing).

If you look at high glycemic foods in the right way, you will see them for the destructive impostors for nutrition that they actually are!

I wish you good success in this process with the confidence that a LCR is an abundantly more healthful and beneficial choice than high glycemic binging!

IV. Low-Carb Potential Benefits in Anti-Aging

1. Decoding Immortality

A recent Smithsonian channel full episode (viewable on your computer via **http://www.smithsonianchannel.com/site/sn/show.do?show=137613**) chronicled the 2009 Nobel Prize research in microbiology that holds the potential to dramatically extend life AND to reverse aging. The down side is that the mechanism activating this panacea may also trigger cancer (after all, the hallmark of cancer is "unrestrained growth").

2. The Hayflick Limit

Fifty years ago Professor Leonard Hayflick – Cell Biologist, UCSF – found that certain cells critical to health, vitality and "anti-aging" can reproduce only fifty times before entering into senescence (cell "old age") and then, ultimately, cell death. This became known as the "Hayflick Limit."

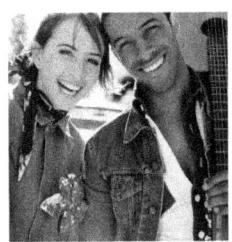 The result is an effective human mortality limit that ensures typically limited life spans of between 80 to 100 years. It also creates the "aging" process in which youth, vitality and health are gradually but irrevocably eroded.

Or are they?

3. Nobel Laureate Elizabeth Blackburn

Nobel laureate Elizabeth Blackburn discovered that when cells replicate, the "ends" of chromosomes (telomeres) are shortened. When they reach "terminal" shortening, cell death is imminent.

An enzyme named telomerase was subsequently discovered. This enzyme is capable of repairing the accumulated damage to telomeres by lengthening them. Theoretically, this would make cells immortal, but – again – the downside is the potential triggering of cancerous growths.

Dr. Blackburn's research is creating an intense search for a drug able to stimulate the production of telomerase within humans. One such drug, called TA-65 is already in clinical trials.

4. Elixir for Life

In the report, **Elixir for Life**, Professor David Sinclair is quick to remind those who seek such drugs of the inherent problem of stimulating cancer. Dr. Sinclair is also ardently in pursuit of a concentrated form of resveratrol which may actually slow aging.

5. A Potential Low-Carb Impact

Dr. Paul Magarelli of the Institute for Sustained Health reports that overcoming insulin resistance – a by-product of a properly adopted LCR – has the potential benefit of overcoming propensity toward cancer, high blood pressure, heart disease and diabetes.

Is there a connection between controlling the cancer triggering aspects of the newly discovered telomerase enzyme as stimulated by drugs like TA-65? Could the keto-genic (keto-lipolysis) metabolism stimulated by an effective LCR overcome the cancer triggering properties of telomerase?

Summarizing Our Efforts To This Point

The LCR is not a diet: We do not diet ("dieting" implies depriving ourselves of eating), we feast up to eight times per day on the most amazingly delicious foods!

The LCR has transformed my life by allowing me to lose (and continue to keep off) 65 pounds without dieting and – more importantly to me – without ever truly being hungry!

My energy level, blood pressure, and lipid levels are all optimized. I am now able to enjoy not only light aerobic exercise but also heavier body building and mountain biking. I'm wearing clothes in sizes I love and I like what I see in the mirror!

Having achieved my Low-Carb Regimen (LCR) goal of 65 pounds lost, I continue to enjoy adding back more vigorous recreational pursuits. As noted above, most recently I have taken up mountain biking and commend this activity to those whose health and interests lead them to pursue it. This is a wonderful way to get exercise and is enjoyed by all ages from the young to those who are more senior in their ages.

With those 65 pounds lost I continue to weigh-in at 179 pounds (plus or minus two pounds depending on whether I'm measuring per my "**having fun getting on the scale**" regimen). I continue to love wearing size 33 inch waist clothes (down from the 48 inch slacks I had to wear before switching to my LCR).

This is my kind of a program: Losing weight and gaining healthful vitality by constantly eating the right kinds of flavourful, nutritious low-carb foods!

It is my hope that – with the help of this book to aid you in implementing the Low-Carb Regimen (LCR) – that your experience will be the same!

Chapter Fifteen
Where's the Test for Insulin Resistance?

I. What is insulin resistance?

1. The Body: A "factory" of cells producing "outcomes"

A simplistic way of viewing the operation of the body is to see it as a "factory" producing "outcomes" enabled by the operation, maintenance and repair of the cells within our body. The successful operation of cells enables thought, motion, emotion, reproduction and other bodily by-products. This amazing "factory" requires fuel for its cells – primarily food (that must be converted to other forms) – in order to have the energy to produce those outcomes. Foods – in turn – are broadly input as carbohydrates, proteins or fats.

2. Fuel for Cells and the Three Treatments of Carbs:

Carbohydrates themselves are generally treated by the body as sugars, starches or fibers. Sugars and starches are readily converted into blood sugar (glucose – the primary form of "fuel" for cell energy) within our blood stream. Fiber is typically not absorbed for these purposes (therefore, fiber is subtracted when counting "net" carbs in our diet – see Chapter Two,

Section V of this book: How to count carbs). Instead, fiber is useful to our bodies in other ways.

3. Carbs Converted to Glucose (fuel for cells) – Transported by Insulin:

The cells in our bodies need to be able to absorb this glucose so that they can convert it into energy to fuel cell operations. To aid in this process our bodies produce insulin which transports the glucose for absorption into our cells.

This amazing process is all very efficient and a marvel of biochemical engineering!

4. Cells Losing Their Ability to Respond to Insulin:

But what happens when we flood our bloodstreams with too much glucose (excess carbs) and/or the cells begin to lose their ability to respond to the insulin (and glucose is not as readily absorbed)?

The typical end result is that the excess glucose is used for "intermediate" storage and then – ultimately – for "long-term" storage throughout our bodies as fat.

5. The Problem of Too Much Glucose and Fat Storage:

To oversimplify, the problem for many is too much glucose from carbs and cells that are losing their ability to absorb that glucose.

It is as if the cells become "weary" of the endless flood of blood sugar from carbohydrates and begin "resisting" it. We still need energy for our cells, but now our cells reject more and more of the glucose from the carbohydrates we consume. The end result is that we store more and more fat.

Our cells are now actually short on the energy they need: We tire more easily and seek more fuel (typically in the form of more carbs) to compensate.

6. Excess Carbs as a Counterproductive Cycle of Fat Production:

A counterproductive cycle has begun: We need more energy so we consume more carbs. This causes us to produce more insulin to aid in transporting the glucose to our cells. However, our cells are now rejecting the "shipment" so we put the shipment into long-term storage (fat).

Said another way, our cells have become resistant to the "shipments" (of glucose) that insulin seeks to deliver.

II. How many people are affected by insulin resistance?

1. Insulin Resistance Is Not as Easily Determined:

Estimates vary on the numbers within our population affected by insulin resistance. Diabetes – a potential outcome of unchecked insulin resistance – and obesity (frequently, but not always, associated with insulin resistance) are more easily determined. It is suggested that anywhere from a quarter to over half of our population either have or will develop insulin resistance (or had insulin resistance and it has now progressed to something more easily recognized).

2. The Epidemic of Obesity:

According to a Feb 10, 2010 report:

"the Gallup-Healthways Well-Being Index showed that 63.1% of adults in the U.S. were either overweight or obese in 2009."

An October 7, 2011 article reported:

"the majority of Americans are still at an unhealthy weight – either overweight or obese (61.6%)."

Another report stated:

"Obesity is more prevalent in the United States than any other country, including other Western industrialized regions like the United Kingdom. And it's not just adults suffering from weight problems – but children and adolescents too! According to the National Institutes of Health, 17% of children and adolescents aged 2 to 19 years were overweight in 2004. And what's more alarming is 32.2% of adults suffer from obesity (that's almost 90 million) – which is a dangerous step up from just being plain overweight. Another 30% of Americans are simply overweight."

Now described as an epidemic, the percentage of Americans overweight or obese has doubled since the 1980s.

3. What Is Obesity?

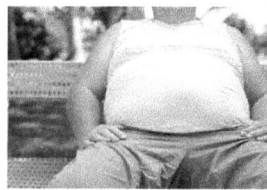

How many of us have stepped onto a Wii Fit platform, input our height and then had the machine – after it has measured our weight – announce, "That's obese!"?

According to the medical dictionary definition of popular terms a person has traditionally been considered to be obese if they are more than 20 percent over their ideal weight. That ideal weight must take into account the person's height, age, sex, and build.

Obesity has been more precisely defined by the National Institutes of Health (the NIH) as a BMI of 30 and above. (A BMI of 30 is about 30 pounds overweight.)

4. The True Danger of Being Obese and Overweight:

The **Medical Dictionary Definition of Popular Terms** goes on to state that being overweight is a significant contributor to health problems. It increases the risk of developing a number of diseases including:

- Type II (adult-onset) diabetes

- High blood pressure (hypertension)

- Stroke (cerebrovascular accident or CVA)

- Heart attack (myocardial infarction or MI)

- Heart failure (congestive heart failure)

- Cancer (certain forms such as cancer of the prostate and cancer of the colon and rectum)

- Gallstones and gall bladder disease (cholecystitis)

- Gout and gouty arthritis

- Osteoarthritis (degenerative arthritis) of the knees, hips, and the lower back

- Sleep apnea (failure to breath normally during sleep, lowering blood oxygen)

- Pickwickian syndrome (obesity, red face, underventilation, and drowsiness).

5. Insulin Resistance Is a Precursor to These Problems:

This is not a trivial problem and a growing body of research is developing around it. One reason for this is that insulin resistance is seen as a pre-diabetic condition – previously identified as a serious and growing health concern.

It should be noted, however, that not all who have insulin resistance are overweight or obese and not all who are overweight or obese are insulin resistant. Having said this, the general trend is that excess body fat – particularly in the form of belly fat among those forty and older – is associated with insulin resistance.

These concerns lead many to seek a test that will determine the presence or absence of insulin resistance.

III. What tests are available for insulin resistance?

1. The Test for Scientific Research (Difficult and Expensive):

There is a scientific procedure – difficult to administer and expensive – that is considered by many as the specific test for insulin resistance: The **Euglycemic clamp**.

2. A Possible Future Test:

A recent research article describes a **new test**. Administration of this test only requires ingestion of a [13C]glucose "marked" solution followed by a breath test. This is certainly quick and easy, but it is not available at this time.

3. The More Commonly Used Tests:

Two more general tests used to indicate insulin resistance are **the fasting glucose test** and **the glucose tolerance test**. Both of these tests require an eight hour period of fasting (not my personal preference). In both tests a blood sugar analysis is then performed. In the glucose tolerance test a strongly sweetened fluid is then ingested and then two hours later another blood sugar analysis is administered for comparative purposes.

4. The A1c Blood Test:

Another general test used is **the A1c blood test**. The A1c test and **eAG** result give a picture of the average amount of glucose in the blood over the last few months.

You will need a qualified health care professional to order these tests, to interpret their results and to provide any requisite health care treatment.

5. The Need to Understand Insulin Resistance:

Most people have never heard of insulin resistance and yet this condition increases the chance of developing type II diabetes and heart disease.

Learning about insulin resistance is the first step toward making lifestyle changes that can help prevent type II diabetes and other health problems.

IV. What are the general "indicators" for insulin resistance?

The following information is taken from the **National Diabetes Information Clearinghouse** (NDIC):

1. General Indicators of Insulin Resistance:

Although insulin resistance may be difficult to routinely determine, there are some general "indicators" (suggestive, but not conclusive in and of themselves) that insulin resistance is in operation:

- Being overweight, especially around the midsection (belly fat)

- Sedentary lifestyle

- Age greater than 40 years

- High blood pressure

- High cholesterol

- Having PCOS (Polycystic Ovarian Syndrome)

- Certain ethnic groups (Hispanic, African American or Native American)

2. When Insulin Resistance Is Suspected:

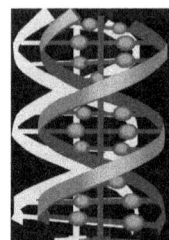 If you meet some of these criteria, your doctor may suspect that you are insulin resistant. The next step is blood testing to look at how well your body deals with sugar. These tests, used to diagnose pre-diabetes or diabetes, include the fasting glucose level and the glucose tolerance test.

Insulin resistance can affect the proportion of the body's lipids, significantly increasing the amount of triglycerides and sdLDLs (small dense lipoproteins) in the blood and decreasing the amount of HDL (high density lipoprotein, the "good cholesterol"). It may also increase a person's risk of developing a blood clot, cause inflammatory changes, and increase a person's sodium retention, which can lead to increased blood pressure.

3. Metabolic Syndrome, Insulin Resistance and Syndrome X:

Many people with insulin resistance and high blood glucose have other conditions that increase the risk of developing type II diabetes and damage to the heart and blood vessels, also called cardiovascular disease. As noted before, these conditions include having excess weight around the waist, high blood pressure, and abnormal levels of cholesterol and triglycerides in the blood. Having several of these problems is called metabolic syndrome or insulin resistance syndrome, formerly called syndrome X.

4. Metabolic Syndrome:

More precisely then, metabolic syndrome (aka "insulin resistance" or "syndrome X") is defined as the presence of any three of the following conditions:

- waist measurement of 40 inches or more for men and 35 inches or more for women

- triglyceride levels of 150 milligrams per deciliter (mg/dL) or above, or taking medication for elevated triglyceride levels

- HDL, or "good," cholesterol level below 40 mg/dL for men and below 50 mg/dL for women, or taking medication for low HDL levels

- blood pressure levels of 130/85 or above, or taking medication for elevated blood pressure levels

- fasting blood glucose levels of 100 mg/dL or above, or taking medication for elevated blood glucose levels

V. A Review of Insulin, Glucose and Insulin Resistance:

The following information is taken from **labtestsonline.org**:

1. Insulin and Glucose Described More Precisely:

Insulin is a hormone produced by the beta cells in the pancreas. Small amounts of it are normally released after each meal to help transport glucose into the body's cells, where it is needed for energy production. Insulin resistance is a decreased ability to respond to the effects of insulin, especially by muscle and fat (adipose) tissues. Since cells must have glucose to survive, the body compensates for insulin resistance by producing additional amounts of the hormone. This results in a state of hyperinsulinemia in the blood and over-stimulation of some tissues that have remained insulin sensitive. Over time, this process causes an imbalance in the relationship between glucose and insulin and can cause an unhealthy ripple effect in the body.

2. Metabolic Syndrome and Insulin Resistance Described More Precisely:

Metabolic syndrome and insulin resistance are two terms that have often been used interchangeably to characterize some of the abnormalities associated with increased resistance to insulin and increased production of insulin, and to recognize these changes as risk factors for future disease. Metabolic syndrome is essentially a subset of insulin resistance, with a focus on identifying obese, sedentary people who are beginning to experience alterations in their lipid levels and impaired glucose processing. The goal of this identification is to work with these people to decrease their health risks through lifestyle changes.

3. The Cause of Insulin Resistance:

The cause of insulin resistance is not fully understood. It is thought to be due partly to genetic factors, including ethnicity, and due partly to lifestyle. Most patients with insulin resistance do not have any symptoms – they do not realize that this process is taking place in their bodies. In most cases, the body is able to keep pace with the need for extra insulin production for many years. If or when the body's insulin production fails to keep up with demand, then hyperglycemia will occur. Once glucose levels reach a high enough level, diabetes is present; the high glucose levels can damage blood vessels in many organs, including the kidneys. Insulin resistance that is associated with these high glucose levels is a risk factor for developing type II diabetes.

Changes in lipids can cause fatty plaque deposits in the arteries and lead to cardiovascular disease and strokes.

Scientists have identified specific genes that make people more likely to develop insulin resistance and diabetes. Again, excess weight and lack of physical activity also contribute to insulin resistance.

As an aside on "specific genes that make people more likely to develop insulin resistance and diabetes," I wonder if the socioeconomic, cultural disposition in our contemporary society to load up on highly refined carbs is more the culprit than "genetics."

I am prompted to this thinking by the work in the early 1900s of Dr. Weston Price. Dr. Price documented dramatic comparisons between siblings where the older family members ate traditional "ancestral" diets but the younger siblings were fed "the foods of commerce" (highly refined carbohydrates): The results were not pretty.

Many people with insulin resistance and high blood glucose have other conditions that increase the risk of developing type 2 diabetes and damage to the heart and blood vessels, also called cardiovascular disease. For emphasis, these conditions include having excess weight around the waist, high blood pressure, and abnormal levels of cholesterol and triglycerides in the blood.

Having several of these problems is called metabolic syndrome or insulin resistance syndrome, formerly called syndrome X.

4. Insulin Resistance Is Not a Disease or a Diagnosis:

According to labtestsonline.org:

Insulin resistance is not a disease or specific diagnosis, but it has been associated with conditions such as cardiovascular disease (CVD), hypertension, polycystic ovarian syndrome (PCOS), type II diabetes, obesity, and non-alcoholic fatty liver disease. Some researchers also believe that there may be a link between insulin resistance and some forms of cancer. The mechanisms of these associations, however, are not well understood. It is important to remember that many of the people who have these conditions do not have insulin resistance and, likewise, many of the people who have insulin resistance will never develop these conditions. These are just patterns of association that have emerged. They are frequently seen together and it is thought that insulin resistance may contribute to their development and exacerbate them when it is present.

VI. What can be done to treat insulin resistance?

1. Diet and Lifestyle Change

Treatment of insulin resistance primarily involves changes in diet and lifestyle. The American Diabetes Association (ADA) recommends losing excess weight, getting regular amounts of moderate-intensity physical activity, and increasing dietary fiber to lower blood insulin levels and increase the body's sensitivity to it.

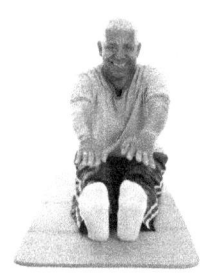

Weight loss and regular exercise can:

- Decrease blood pressure levels

- Increase insulin sensitivity

- Decrease triglyceride and LDL levels

- Raise HDL levels

2. Not All "Diet and Lifestyle Change" Plans Are Equal:

The "Food Pyramid" of the past promoted a high carb, low-fat diet.

Heart disease, high blood pressure and obesity have sky rocketed since.

On the other hand – at least in my experience – the Low-Carb Regimen (we do NOT diet, we feast! – see in this book: **Foods You Can Eat RIGHT Now, Beverages You Can Drink Right Now** and **Where's**

My Bread?) may aid our bodies in switching from a body-fat accumulating cycle to a fat-burning cycle. These sections of this book and the section dealing with, **why you should crave a fat burning metabolism**, provide a more detailed description of how this process works.

3. An Insulin Resistance Medical Practitioner:

Patients who are identified by their doctors as having insulin resistance should work with their doctor and with other medical professionals, such as a nutritionist, to develop an individualized treatment plan and to monitor its effectiveness. Drug treatments may also be necessary to control any existing, underlying, associated conditions and diseases.

Chapter Fifteen Conclusion:

So, where's the test for insulin resistance?

As explained in this chapter, there is no simple across-the-counter test available (as there is for measuring the body's production of ketones) – see:

How to Know If You Are Really Burning Fat (by measuring ketones)

As also explained, there are clearly visible and readily identifiable "conditions" associated with insulin resistance, not the least of which is excess belly fat.

Go ahead: Pinch the flab around your belly (most of us have it).

Wouldn't you be better off without it? And wouldn't it be more fun to lose it if you weren't hungry in the process?

If your answer is "Yes!," then you may want to consider – if you have not already done so – applying the Low-Carb Regimen described in this book!

Sample Menu Guidelines

*You may wish to **Return to the Introductory Menu***

*Or go to the **Brief Table of Contents***

Keep in mind that we count net grams of carbs, not calories. Accordingly, for Step One in our Low-Carb Regimen (LCR), our goal is 60 to 80 net grams of carbs daily. In Steps Two through Four our goal is just 50 net grams of carbs. In Step Five we may increase our carb intake – perhaps to 80, or more, net grams of carbs daily – so long as it does not interfere with the maintenance of our weight loss.

The ideas presented in this book are key to the effectiveness of a menu, such as the Sample Menu listed below. In a low-carb regimen, we focus on high protein, high healthful fat, low-carb foods. Failure to embrace the low-carb regimen – in other words eating high carb along with high fat and high protein foods – could be a prescription for disaster.

Low-carb leftovers are wonderful anytime we need a feast!

Below are some ideas for feasting selections, but there are countless options. Just be sure that the original food from which you take your leftover is truly low-carb!

Low-carb Leftover Options:

- slices of roast beef

- slices of pork

- low-carb fried chicken

- a slice of omelet

- a slice of egg strata

- a slice of low-carb cheesecake

- a slice of low-carb pumpkin pie

- a tasty salad

*Of course, it is not necessary to eat **all** of the food listed in the "Sample Menu!"*

Instead, we eat when we actually are hungry (up to eight meals per day). Foods consumed, however, must be low-carb: Read the labels carefully and follow the guidelines in this book!

Note: As a result of being able to eat up to eight meals per day we do not suffer the ongoing "hunger" discomfort of other weight-loss approaches.

A side benefit is that as we eat smaller, more frequent meals our stomachs painlessly shrink. Needing smaller portions to feel full also helps us maintain our weight loss as we progress through The Five Steps of the Low-Carb Regimen (LCR).

In addition, any of the foods from The 1 to 5 Low-Carb Cooking Guide at the end of this book may be used to substitute for items in the Sample Menu, above. Obviously selecting Relatively Low-Carb Cheesecake for eight meals in your day is going to deprive you of the more balanced nutrition that comes from the variety built into the Sample 1st Week Menu! Also, per the cheesecake title, it is only relatively low-carb.

Note: Processed foods - such as Nathan's wieners - may have nutritional drawbacks such as the inclusion of nitrates and nitrites. Organic options are available. However, Nathan's wieners are low-carb, tasty and easily obtained when I want a hotdog (without the bun, of course!).

Keep in mind also the **Foods Eaten Up To Eight Times Per Day** from Chapter Four, the **Beverages To Drink** from Chapter Twelve, the **Foods To Eat** from Chapter Thirteen, and – of course – the **1 To 5 Cooking Guide** at the back of this book.

Sample One Week Menu

Day One thru Seven: Pre-Breakfast

- Food supplements

- Low-carb protein or whey shake

- coffee, tea, infused-water or unsweetened, unflavored coconut milk latte

Breakfast

Day One:

- 2 fried eggs
- 3 strips of bacon
- 1/8 avocado with a dollop of low-carb sour cream
- 2 strawberries
- coffee, tea, infused-water or unsweetened, unflavored coconut milk latte

Day Two:

- a delectable cheese and sautéed Bell pepper, onion and celery omelet
- 3 strips of bacon
- 1/8 avocado with a dollop of low-carb sour cream
- 2 strawberries
- coffee, tea, infused-water or unsweetened, unflavored coconut milk latte

Day Three:

- a slice of egg strata
- a breakfast salad with strawberries and/or blueberries

- coffee, tea, infused-water or unsweetened, unflavored coconut milk latte

Day Four:

- scrambled eggs with shreds of Cheddar cheese

- 3 strips of bacon

- a breakfast salad with strawberries and/or blueberries

- coffee, tea, infused-water or unsweetened, unflavored coconut milk latte

Day Five:

- a delectable cheese and sautéed Bell pepper, onion and celery omelet

- a breakfast salad with strawberries and/or blueberries

- coffee, tea, infused-water or unsweetened, unflavored coconut milk latte

Day Six:

- low-carb pancakes with butter and low-carb maple syrup

- 2 fried eggs

- 3 strips of bacon

- 1/8 avocado with a dollop of low-carb sour cream

- 2 strawberries

- coffee, tea, infused-water or unsweetened, unflavored coconut milk latte

Day Seven:

- a slice of egg strata

- 1/8 avocado with a dollop of low-carb sour cream

- 2 strawberries

- coffee, tea, infused-water or unsweetened, unflavored coconut milk latte

Day One thru Seven: 2nd-Breakfast

- 1 string cheese

- 1 pkg Emerald Dry Roasted Almonds

- and/or Bell pepper slices

- and/or celery with blueberry embedded cream cheese

- coffee, tea, infused-water or unsweetened, unflavored coconut milk latte

Day One thru Seven: Lunch

- lunch salad

- low-carb leftovers (perhaps, slices of roast beef or fried chicken!)

  - *Note:* *When I'm in a hurry or just in the mood, I like to bring two Nathan's wieners and a couple of dill pickle spears as a replacement for the low-carb leftovers!*

- pre-cooked bacon slices

- a slice of cheddar cheese

- Splenda-jello cup

- Carbmaster yogurt

- coffee, tea, infused-water or unsweetened, unflavored coconut milk latte

Day One thru Seven: 2nd Lunch

- 2 peanut or almond protein balls

- and/or 1 pumpkin protein slice

- and/or Bell pepper slices

- and/or celery with blueberry embedded cream cheese

- coffee, tea, infused-water or unsweetened, unflavored coconut milk latte

Dinner

Day One:

- filleted chicken breast with spinach, bacon, parmesan diced tomatoes
- asparagus with cheese sauce dusted with blue cheese
- Carbmaster yogurt, berry, whipped cream chocolate parfait
- coffee, tea, infused-water or unsweetened, unflavored coconut milk latte

Day Two:

- butter-fried, seasoned lamb chops
- broccoli with my world class cheese sauce
- dinner salad with cucumbers, Bell peppers, avocado, berries and feta cheese!
- Splenda jello with low-carb whipped cream
- coffee, tea, infused-water or unsweetened, unflavored coconut milk latte

Day Three:

- Mission small fajita Carb Control tortilla tacos with Romaine lettuce, sliced grape tomatoes, shredded Cheddar cheese, sour cream and low-carb guacamole

- a small dish of blueberries with low-carb whipped cream

- Cinnamon dusted, butter-fried low-carb tortilla strips

- coffee, tea, infused-water or unsweetened, unflavored coconut milk latte

Day Four:

- butter-fried salmon!

- dinner salad with cucumbers, Bell peppers, avocado, berries and Parmesan cheese!

- sautéed stir-fried onions, Bell peppers and celery dusted with Parmesan cheese

- Carbmaster yogurt, berry, whipped cream chocolate parfait

- coffee, tea, infused-water or unsweetened, unflavored coconut milk latte

Day Five:

- Zoupa Tuscana

- low-carb tortilla rollups

- dinner salad with cucumbers, Bell peppers, avocado, berries and feta cheese!

- a small dish of blueberries with (or without) low-carb cream

- coffee, tea, infused-water or unsweetened, unflavored coconut milk latte

Day Six:

- Low-carb fried chicken with bacon and blue cheese crumbles

- asparagus with cheese sauce dusted with blue cheese

- Splenda jello topped with low-carb whipping cream

- coffee, tea, infused-water or unsweetened, unflavored coconut milk latte

Day Seven:

- slow-crocked pork roast

- butter sautéed green beans

- slices of cheddar cheese

- dill pickle spears

- low-carb pumpkin pie with whipped cream

- coffee, tea, infused-water or unsweetened, unflavored coconut milk latte

Post-Dinner

In addition to our usual selections such as:

- 1 pkg Emerald Dry Roasted Almonds

- and/or Bell pepper slices

- and/or celery with blueberry embedded cream cheese

- and/or decaffeinated latte

- and/or iced tea

- and/or infused water

For variety, consider:

Day One:

- Splenda-jello with whipped cream

Day Two:

- Carbmaster yogurt topped with a tbsp of low-carb whipped cream and sprinkles of low-carb (bakers) cocoa

Day Three:

- celery with cream cheese, or Cheddar cheese, or peanut or almond butter

Day Four:

- a slice of honeydew melon

Day Five:

- a slice of watermelon

Day Six:

- Carbmaster yogurt topped with a tbsp of low-carb whipped cream and sprinkles of low-carb (bakers) cocoa

Day Seven:

- celery with cream cheese, or Cheddar cheese, or peanut or almond butter

1 to 5 - Low-Carb Cooking Guide

I. A Sample Low-Carb Meal

Entrée:

We had filleted chicken breast layered with Italian seasonings, sesame seeds, fresh spinach, and bacon strips covered in marinara sauce and liberally sprinkled with a parmesan and Romano cheese blend. The chicken fillets were baked in a Pyrex cooking dish lightly coated in olive oil. A small quantity of water was added between the fillets in order to promote moisture retention and uniformity of cooking temperature.

Side:

The fillets were served with freshly cooked asparagus sautéed in butter and garnished with a made from scratch cheddar sauce comprised of butter, milled flax seed, a little milk and grated sharp cheddar cheese.

Beverages:

I drank fresh lime infused water while my spouse drank vanilla flavoured almond milk.

Dessert:

King Soopers Carbmaster vanilla yogurt garnished with fresh, sliced strawberries. We were too full from dinner and had to wait a while to eat dessert.

(The detailed recipe for this meal is contained in the "Recipes" section of this "Cooking Guide.")

The aroma, the texture and the flavour of the meal were indescribably delicious and satisfying!

II. Suggested External Cookbooks

Lo-Carb Cookbook: 6 Ingredients, 6 Easy Steps

**Low-carb and Gluten Free Comfort Foods –
Recipes to Keep You Going**

Recipes

III. True Low-Carb Flax Seed Yeast Bread

1. Preheat your oven to 425 degrees Fahrenheit.

2. Beat 1 egg in a mixing bowl.

3. Combine with the beaten egg in the mixing bowl:

- 1/2 cups of CarbQuik – 3 grams of carbs

- 1/2 cup of Carbalose – 9 grams of carbs

- 2 tablespoons of coconut flour – 4 grams of carbs

- 1/2 teaspoon of sea salt

- 1 tablespoon of milled flax seeds

- 1 teaspoon of granulated sugar – about 4 grams of carbs

*Real sugar is needed for proper yeast action

Note: The non-sugar, artificial sweeteners do not appear to allow yeast to function correctly (some actually appear to impede the yeast action). Although sugar is high carbohydrate and high glycemic, the amount of the sugar is sufficiently low to keep both the total carb count and the glycemic impact low per slice of this bread.

Per the Livestrong website:

"Refined sugar is composed entirely of carbohydrates. One teaspoon, or 4.2 grams of sugar, contains 4.2 grams of carbohydrates."

"Brown sugar is slightly more diet-friendly than white sugar. At 11 calories per teaspoon, brown sugar contains 2.9 grams of carbohydrates."

To read more: See **How Many Calories Are There In Sugar?**

4. In 1/3 cup of warm water (of a separate measuring cup) mix:

- 1 teaspoon of granulated sugar – about 4 grams of carbs

- 2 packets of Hodgson Mills yeast for whole grain breads

5. Blend the yeast, sugar, water from the measuring cup into the mixing bowl flours and beaten egg.

6. Add 1/2 cup of unsweetened, unflavoured coconut milk into the measuring cup that contained the yeast-sugar-water mixture.

7. Warm (do not boil) the coconut milk in your microwave.

8. Melt two tablespoons of butter and mix into the warmed unsweetened, unflavoured coconut milk. (about 1 gram of carbs)

9. Blend the butter - unsweetened, unflavored coconut milk mixture into the mixing bowl containing the flours, egg and sugar-water-yeast.

Note: Your mixture will have a texture similar to oatmeal cookie dough. Do not attempt to "work" the dough as you would a traditional bread dough.

10. Spray canola oil on the inside of a Pyrex loaf pan.

11. Use a spatula to scrape the dough into the Pyrex loaf pan.

12. Let the dough rise in a warm place for about one half hour.

13. Sprinkle 1/2 teaspoon of milled flax seeds over the top of the risen bread.

14. Bake at 425 degrees Fahrenheit for 20 to 25 minutes. Adjust baking time in accordance with your elevation and oven performance. The bread will smell done and will have a light golden colour to its top and sides.

15. Let the baked bread sit and cool in the Pyrex loaf pan for 15 minutes. Then use a thin butter knife to ensure the sides of the loaf have separated from the walls of the loaf pan. Place a small cutting board or plate over the top of the loaf pan and "turn the bread out" onto the cutting board or plate.

After the bread is turned out, spread butter lightly across the crust of the bread and allow this to "settle in" while the bread continues to cool.

The bread will cut into 12 to 20 slices of varying thickness. The bread has a nice texture and sticks together well even in very thin slices. The bread also has that wonderful "true yeast" flavour and aroma that we tend to lose out on when we eat low-carb. Since there are only about 26 grams of carbs in the entire loaf, each slice is no more than 2 1/2 grams of carbs. This is a wonderful low-carb count since most store bought breads have more carbs per slice than the true low-carb flax seed yeast bread has in an entire loaf!

I suggest serving the bread with lots of butter. As noted above, it is delicious, nutritious, low-carb and high fiber!

IV. New York Style Baked Cheesecake, Version One

See recipe VI for version two!

A. Create an almond flour, melted butter, granulated Stevia cake "crust"

1. Preheat your oven to 425 degrees Fahrenheit.

2. Place four tablespoons of butter (Challenge butter or another cream-rich butter is suggested) in a medium sized, deep-dish Pyrex cake dish (mine is about 8 by 11 inches on top and slants down slightly on the sides).

Then place the Pyrex cake dish with the butter in the oven until the butter is mostly melted. This should only take a few minutes.

3. Remove the cake dish with the melted butter and rotate the cake dish (with kitchen gloves!) to make sure the butter is spread evenly across the bottom of the cake dish.

4. Then spread 1/2 cup of almond flour (actually, almond "flour" is a "meal" that is merely called a flour!) over the butter.

5. Sprinkle 1/4 cup of granulated Stevia over the almond flour and spread the butter, almond flour, and granulated Stevia around with a fork.

6. Pat the mixture evenly across the bottom of the cake dish with a flat spatula.

7. Place the cake dish into the oven and bake for 15 to 20 minutes until a toasted golden brown. Keep in mind that this crust is NOT a traditional white flour crust. Instead it is more like a light graham cracker crust (without the carbs). Heads up: This crust will smell unbelievably delicious as it nears its toasted golden to medium brown perfection!

8. Remove the cake dish from the oven when it is done and allow it to cool before adding the New York style cheesecake filling.

B. Create your New York style cheesecake filling

1. Beat four fresh eggs (I like Egglands Best) in a mixing bowl.

2. Mix in 1/2 cup of Stevia granulated sweetener and 1/2 teaspoon sea salt.

3. Mix in 1/2 cup of CarbQuik flour.

4. Mix in one 16-ounce container of fat rich sour cream (do NOT use reduced fat sour cream!).

5. Add in two 8-ounce packages of regular cream cheese (I like the Philadelphia brand). Again, do not use reduced fat varieties!

6. Use a fork and a knife to cut and blend the cream cheese into the egg, flour, Stevia, sea salt and sour cream mixture.

7. Cut a lemon in half and pick out the seeds. Squeeze all of the juice from the lemon into the mixing bowl mixture.

Note: The secret to really good New York style cheesecake is the right balance between the sour cream, the lemon and the sweetener. Adjust these until you get the flavour that suits you. My recipe is just right for me!

8. Blend the ingredients thoroughly together until mostly smooth - there will be small, cream cheese "lumps" in your mixture.

C. Combining and Finishing

1. Pour the blended cream cheese filling into the cooled cake dish.

2. Bake the cheesecake in your pre-heated oven at 425 degrees Fahrenheit for about 30 minutes. You will know it is done by the golden brown on its sides and by the signs of browning (caramelization) on top. In addition the cheesecake will rise somewhat in the middle and this will create some "cracks" in its surface. The "cracks" will collapse back into the surface of the cheesecake as it cools.

3. Allow the baked cheesecake to cool at least one hour.

4. Refrigerate overnight.

I like to serve this cheesecake just as it is. Some like to serve it with whipped cream and strawberries.

It really is extraordinary: Enjoy!

V. Delicious Low-Carb Clam Chowder

Zoupa Tuscana version:

The following soup can also be made with low-carb chicken broth and mild Italian Sausage (hot – if you like spicy!) in place of the clam juice and the clams. In addition, replace the broccoli with 1 cup of kale (I also eliminate the Xanthan gum) and the result is similar to the Olive Garden's Sausage and Kale (Zoupa Tuscana) soup.

1. Melt two tablespoons of butter in a soup pan.

2. Add:

- ¼ chopped onion
- ½ cup chopped broccoli (frozen works fine – microwave to soften before chopping)
- ½ cup chopped celery
- Sauté to preference

3. Add:

- 1 10-ounce can of baby clams (include the juice from the can!)

*For extra flavour, add one 8-ounce bottle of clam juice, too

4. Warm (do not boil) in a 2 cup Pyrex measuring cup in a microwave:

- 8 ounces of half and half cream with an additional

- 8 ounces of unsweetened, unflavored coconut milk

- Mix in with a fork: 1 tsp of Xanthan gum (more or less: depending on how thick you like your chowder)

5. Blend the Pyrex measuring cup contents into the soup pan vegetables

6. Add:

- Liberal grinds of freshly ground black pepper (perhaps 1 tbsp, per your preference)

- ¼ tsp of sea salt

- ¼ tsp of Worcestershire Sauce

- ¼ tsp of garlic powder

- 1 tsp of chopped chives

- 2 tsps of chopped parsley

- 10 drops of liquid Stevia and gently stir while simmering

7. Add: 8 more ounces of unsweetened, unflavoured coconut milk

8. Heat until desired serving temperature

Note: Taste and see if the flavouring is satisfying and add more seasonings as needed. If any flavour is too strong, add more unsweetened, unflavoured coconut milk and, again, adjust your seasonings.

Serving Suggestion:

I like to serve this soup with my relatively low-carb biscuits topped with butter. I add a wonderful side salad and finish off with low-carb orange jello topped with whipping cream. What a delicious, nutritious and satisfying feast!

VI. Low-Carb New York Style Cheesecake, Version Two

Let's look, again, at one of my favourite low-carb foods: Low-Carb New York Style Cheesecake.

Version Two has slight variations from Versions One. I encourage experimenting with recipes!

The secret to New York Style Cheesecake is the wonderful tangy flavour that comes from the contrast between good cream cheese and good sour cream. For best results, do not skimp on the quality and fat content of either of these key ingredients. Also, the contrast between these flavours is subtle: Do not overwhelm this subtlety with either too much lemon or too much sweetener.

1. Creating the cheesecake crust

- Pre-heat your oven to 425 degrees (Fahrenheit).

- Place four tablespoons of butter in a medium sized Pyrex dish and let the butter melt (but not burn) by heating the dish with the butter in your oven.

- Remove the dish from the oven and spread ½ cup of almond flour across the floor of the Pyrex dish. I like to use a fork for this.

- Sprinkle ¼ cup of granulated Stevia over the almond flour and use the fork to thoroughly mix the almond flour, melted butter and the Stevia.

- Then use the fork to distribute the mixture evenly across the floor of the Pyrex dish. I like to use a flat spatula to "even out" the mixture so that it is flat, uniformly distributed, and so that there are no unfilled spaces on the floor of my Pyrex dish.

- Place the dish back in the oven and allow the almond flour crust to bake until a "tan" color forms.

- Remove from the oven and allow to cool.

2. Creating the cheesecake filling

- Add two raw eggs to a mixing bowl and whip with a fork

- Blend two 8 ounce packages of Philadelphia brand original cream cheese along with 8 ounces of rich (full fat, please!) sour cream into the whipped eggs.

- Mix in ¼ cup of Stevia and ½ cup of coconut flour.

- Add in 1 cup of unsweetened, unflavoured coconut milk

- Add in the whites of two eggs.

- Blend this mixture until smooth.

- Mix in lemon flavoring to suit (this depends greatly on the kind of lemon flavoring used – experiment until you get it the way you like it!).

- Pour the mixture into the almond "crusted" Pyrex dish.

3. Baking and cooling the cheesecake

- Bake at 425 degrees (Fahrenheit) for 30 to 40 minutes.

- Turn off the oven and allow the mixture to bake and cool for another 30 minutes.

Note: The center of the cheesecake (before sitting the extra 30 minutes in the oven) tends to jiggle. It will firm up as it sets and cools.

- Remove from the oven and allow to set for one hour.

- Place in the refrigerator for at least one hour.

VII. Low-Carb Biscuits and Gravy for Breakfast

Note: This is a favourite breakfast meal for many parts of the USA. Those who have cultural and/or faith-based opposition to these foods will – of course – avoid them.

Breakfast this morning was a biscuit and sausage gravy topped with two eggs over easy. The biscuits are relatively low-carb baking powder, coconut flour, an egg and coconut milk. The gravy for the biscuit is made with Jimmy Dean Pure Pork sausage to which I add unsweetened, unflavoured coconut milk thickened with a teaspoon of Xanthan gum.

1. Cooking the Sausage with Its Gravy

- I warmed (do not overheat) 2 cups of unsweetened, unflavored coconut milk in the microwave. I then sprinkled 1 teaspoon of Xanthan gum onto the surface of the warmed coconut milk and thoroughly blended the mixture together with a fork.

- I added this mixture into the non-stick frying pan containing my already cooked and crumbled breakfast sausage.

- Stirring this mixture over a medium-low heat, I seasoned it with freshly ground pepper, chives and parsley.

- Add more unflavored, unsweetened coconut milk if a less thick gravy is desired. Simply simmer the gravy longer if a thicker gravy is desired.

2. Making the "Relatively" Low-Carb Biscuit Dough

- Whip 1 egg in a bowl

- Blend in ½ cup of unsweetened unflavored coconut milk (more, if needed)

- Add 3/4 cup of CarbQuik flower with 2 tablespoons of Coconut flour into the bowl

- Blend in 1/8 teaspoon of salt, 1 tablespoons of baking powder and 2 tablespoons of Stevia

3. Making the "Relatively" Low-Carb Biscuit Dough into Biscuits

Note: The dough will be the consistency of an oatmeal cookie mixture. Spoon the dough into the muffin pan openings.

- "Grease" with butter a large muffin pan

- Fill each location about one half to two thirds full

- Bake at 425 degrees for about 20 minutes or until done

Holiday Recipes and Thoughts

When it is time for the holidays, here are some low-carb foods that you can enjoy!

VIII. Fresh Pumpkin Spice Egg Nog

This is FRESH egg nog (made with raw eggs) so you will want to drink this within twenty-four hours of its preparation. Also, good quality eggs that are as close to freshly gathered as is feasible are recommended. I live in a larger city, but find Large Egglands Best Eggs used within a few days of purchase adequate.

- Crack 6 fresh eggs into a bowl (I like glass mixing bowls).

- Add ¼ cup of granulated Stevia and whip the eggs and sweetener thoroughly.

- Add 1 ½ cups of unsweetened, unflavored coconut milk.

- Add ½ cup of (liquid) heavy whipping cream and, again, whip the mixture thoroughly.

Now for the fun!

Flavourings are really up to you, but here is what I use for my Fresh Pumpkin Spice Eggnog:

- 2 teaspoons of vanilla

- 1 ½ tablespoons of pumpkin pie spice

- Up to this point I have whipped my mixture with a wire whisk. Now I use my Cuisinart Immersion Blender and thoroughly blend my mixture.

- Cover and place in a cold, non-freezer part of your refrigerator for at least an hour.

- Ladle the mixture into glass mugs and dust lightly with freshly ground nutmeg.

WOW! This eggnog is so good: Flavourful, low-carb, high protein, high fat – just what the low-carb eating regimen doctor ordered!

Options: You could use freshly ground cloves, Vietnamese cinnamon, freshly ground nutmeg or Allspice in any combination to suit.

Some will want to add rum flavouring to suit (real rum is loaded with sugary carbs).

Also, this mixture gets better with refrigeration for about the first 20 hours. The concern in storing fresh eggnog for longer time periods is the bacteria associated with eggs. This is the reason why store-bought eggnogs are loaded with preservatives (not to mention high carb sweeteners, food colourings, thickening agents and various other chemicals).

My wife inquired about thickening the recipe (this mixture is just right for me!). A thicker beverage will result from using all (or, more) heavy whipping cream instead of mostly unflavoured, unsweetened coconut milk (my recipe is three parts coconut milk to one part heavy whipping cream). However, the result will be much higher in carbohydrates.

IX. Pumpkin Spice Eggnog Latte

I prepared my latte as usual:

- 2 measures of freshly ground espresso coffee beans in my 15 bar latte machine – after processing the result is a delicious double shot of espresso.

- 1 ½ cups of steamed and frothed unsweetened, unflavored coconut milk.

- Now, I garnish my latte with a few ounces of the Fresh Pumpkin Spice Eggnog – fabulous!

X. Fresh Whole Berry Orange Cranberry Relish

You'll need a food processor that chops/coarse grinds for this recipe. Alternately, you can chop by hand (but hand-chopping is a lot of work on this particular preparation).

- Freeze one bag of whole cranberries.

- Add the cranberries to your food processor and coarse grind/chop them. Turn off the processor.

- Add 1/3 cup of granulated Stevia into the still off processor.

- Add ½ of a quartered Navel orange – yep, rind and all, so wash the orange thoroughly first – to the blender (only Navel oranges are recommended for this recipe).

- Coarse grind/chop until the orange and Stevia are worked throughout the mixture. Do NOT over-process: The mixture should be somewhat chunky, but not smooth or liquefied. Aim for the consistency of chunky salsa or relish.

- Chill in your refrigerator at least one hour and then serve: Delicious!

Note: Additional Stevia may be added to suit depending on how sweet or tart you like your cranberry relish. It goes without saying that this is delicious with turkey!

XI. Unbelievably Easy Low-Carb Lemon Cheesecake

Here are some quick thoughts on a delicious low-carb dessert that will blow your socks off and – should you share it with others – make you a big hit!

An overview of the process is:

- One: Create the pie crust

- Two: Create the cheesecake filling

- Three: Combine and finish the cheesecake

The detailed instructions follow:

A. Create an almond flour, melted butter, granulated Stevia pie "crust"

1. Preheat your oven to 350 degrees

2. Place three tablespoons of butter (Challenge butter or another cream-rich butter is suggested) in a Pyrex pie dish. Then place the Pyrex pie dish with the butter in the oven until the butter is mostly melted. This should only take a few minutes.

3. Remove the pie dish with the melted butter and rotate the pie dish (with kitchen gloves!) to make sure the butter is spread evenly across the bottom of the pie dish.

4. Then spread 1/2 cup of almond flour (actually, almond "flour" is a "meal" that is merely called a flour!) over the the butter.

5. Sprinkle 1/4 cup of granulated Stevia over the almond flour and spread the butter, almond flour, and granulated Stevia around with a fork.

6. Pat the mixture evenly across the bottom of the pie dish with a flat spatula.

7. Place the pie dish into the oven and bake for 15 to 20 minutes until a toasted golden brown. Keep in mind that this crust is NOT a traditional white flour crust. Instead it is more like a light graham cracker crust (without the carbs). Heads up: This crust will smell unbelievably delicious as it nears its toasted golden brown perfection!

8. Remove from the oven when done and allow to cool before adding the lemon cheesecake filling.

B. Create your lemon, cheesecake filling

1. Use 1 or 2 8-ounce packages of cream cheese (I like the Philadelphia brand) depending on how "deep" you want your cheesecake to fill your pie dish.

2. Place the cream cheese in a sufficiently large mixing bowl.

3. Add 1 package of UNSWEETENED lemon Jello (I like the actual "Jello" brand) for each 8-ounce package of cream cheese.

4. Add 1/4 cup of granulated Stevia for each 8-ounce package of cream cheese.

5. Add 1/2 cup of unsweetened, unflavored coconut milk for each 8-ounce package of cream cheese. More unsweetened, unflavored coconut milk may be added if you desire a "fluffier" filling.

6. Blend the ingredients thoroughly together (until smooth).

C. Combining and Finishing

1. Pour the blended cream cheese filling into the cooled pie dish.

2. Spread the mixture out with a spatula.

3. Garnish with the grated peel of an entire lemon (just the outer yellow portion of the peel – not the white rind). Of course, you will want to wash the lemon thoroughly before grating the peel.

4. Refrigerate for at least an hour.

Warning: This dessert is so delicious that you will find it hard to keep from eating all of it! Even though it is low-carb, over-eating this (or, any) dessert may prove detrimental to your weight-loss goals . . .

The unsweetened Jello is available in lime, orange and several other flavours. I suggest experimenting!

XII. Pumpkin Protein Shake

Although traditional pumpkin pie tends to be packed with carbs (as a result of a flour crust and a cup and a half of sugar added in many recipes!), a low-carb, crustless pumpkin protein pie is a great and flavourful alternative.

A scoop of this pie added to a whey protein shake makes a truly delicious "pumpkin protein shake." I like to dust mine with additional fresh nutmeg and Vietnamese cinnamon!

Alternately – if you do not have any "crustless pumpkin protein pie" on hand, simply open a can of pure pumpkin and add ¼ cup of the pumpkin to your shake.

The rest of the pumpkin from the can refrigerates well when transferred to an appropriate storage container.

XIII. Parmesan Bacon Chicken Strips with Herbs

Fry your fresh chicken strips in a small quantity of olive oil. Add freshly ground pepper and sea salt to taste. Sprinkle fresh herbs. I like the "Simon and Garfunkel" herbs from my wife's garden: Parsley, sage, rosemary and thyme. Turn the strips when the chicken is sufficiently caramelized (browned). Place shreds of pre-cooked bacon strips on the chicken strips. Sprinkle liberally with Parmesan cheese. Serve when cooked to suit: Delicious and nutritious!

XIV. Tangy Deviled Eggs

Cut the hard boiled egg lengthwise and "bend" out the hardened egg yellow into a small dish. For each two eggs that you are "deviling," combine the yellows with 1 tablespoon of softened butter, ½ teaspoon of Stevia, ½ teaspoon of apple cider vinegar and 1 teaspoon of low-carb mustard. Spoon the mixture back into the solid egg white "shells," sprinkle with sea salt, freshly ground pepper and paprika to taste (or, not at all) and enjoy!

1. Hard Boiled Eggs

Store bought, pre-prepared hard boiled eggs are relatively inexpensive although not nearly as good as homemade. Alternately, we can just make our own by the conventional means of boiling them in a pot of water.

2. Egg Cookers

It's not that difficult to boil a pot of water (at least 2 to 3 inches of water) and then add the eggs to be boiled (about 17 minutes for hard boiled, depending on your elevation and the salt content – I add salt – of your water). If you are boiling fresh eggs taken from your refrigerator, it is a good idea to run these eggs under warm water that you gradually increase to hot to help minimize broken egg shells when the eggs are introduced to the boiling water on your stove. I like to use metal tongs to gently place the eggs in the boiling water in order to eliminate cracking that might occur if the eggs sink too rapidly.

Stand alone egg cooking appliances are also available. One inexpensive model is the Home Image Egg Cooker from amazon.com.

XV. Crustless Pumpkin Protein Slices

1. Combine 4 beaten eggs with:

- one large can of pumpkin

- 1 scoop of low-carb whey protein powder
- 4 teaspoons of pumpkin pie spice
- 1 teaspoon of Vietnamese cinnamon
- ¼ cup of granulated Stevia
- ½ cup of unsweetened/unflavored coconut milk
- ¼ cup of half and half cream
- ½ teaspoon of vanilla
- 1 teaspoon of powdered guar gum
- 1 teaspoon of powdered Xanthan gum
- 2 tablespoons of coconut flour
- ¼ teaspoon of salt

2. Mix thoroughly

Note: If you are soy intolerant, watch out for "hidden" soy in whey protein powders. Be particularly cognizant of plant proteins and amino acids. Descriptors beginning with "gluta" and "hydrolyzed" may need closer attention!

Pour the mixture into two separate nine inch round baking dishes that you have sprayed with non-stick oil and then bake at 350 degrees for 30 to 40 minutes (depending on your oven and elevation) or until cooked to your preference.

3. Cool and chill.

4. Serve with whipped topping! Wow!!

XVI. Peanut Protein Balls

Combine:

- ¼ cup of low-carb (read the labels!) chunky peanut butter

- ¼ cup of almond butter

Mix in:

- ¼ cup of almond flour

- ½ teaspoon of vanilla

- 1 scoop of low-carb whey protein powder

(read the labels and watch our for soy if you are allergic to it!)

Note: Moisture content in peanut butter varies greatly. If your mixture is too crumbly, add a little half and half cream until the mixture reaches the desired consistency. The mixture should stick together when a portion of it is rolled into a ball in your hands. In addition, the outside of the "ball" should be shiny and just a little oily from the peanut butter.

Scoop:

Use a tablespoon to scoop out portions of your mixture for rolling into balls.

Roll:

Roll the balls in a small amount of granulated Stevia until each ball is coated.

Roll again:

Then roll the balls in some bakers cocoa.

As noted before, they end up tasting like an American candy: Reese's Peanut Butter Cups.

Freeze:

These bad boys are best really cold!

XVII. World Class Low-Carb Cheese Sauce

- Melt 1 tablespoon of butter in a sauté pan warmed to a medium low heat.

- Blend in two ounces of unwhipped heavy whipping cream

- Blend in ½ cup (or more!) of shredded cheddar cheese

- Blend in fresh rosemary, sage and thyme to taste

To make this sauce extra unbelievably delicious, sprinkle blue cheese crumbles on the items to be garnished with the World Class Low-Carb Cheese Sauce.

I have used this on freshly cooked asparagus, on butter-fried slices of a mesquite smoked pork arm roast, and on fried boneless sesame and pepper seasoned chicken thighs. In all three cases the blending of flavours with the cheese sauce and the blue cheese crumbles was simply extraordinary!

XVIII. Watercress, Avocado and Sliced Strawberry Salad

The ingredients for this salad are in the description. I found fresh watercress at Sunflower Farmer's Markets and I added freshly ground pepper and grape tomatoes to my portion of this salad. You might want to try drizzling a little olive oil and red wine vinegar on this light side-dish. Small portions also make a great garnish on a plate for a larger meal!

XIX. Bacon Avocado Chicken Spinach Romaine and Strawberry Salad

For lunch today I enjoyed some left over chicken in a fresh romaine and spinach salad. I included in the salad avocado, sliced strawberries, freshly ground pepper, shreds of pre-cooked bacon and blue cheese crumbles. For a dressing I sprinkled olive oil and red wine vinegar. It was astonishingly delicious. (If you're not a blue cheese fan, feta, parmesan, pepper jack, or some other cheese of your choice will work fine!)

XX. Gingered Bok Choy, Chicken, Sesame Seed, Bacon Stir Fry

The title for this stir fry reveals the ingredients. I like to begin with some butter in a Teflon pan warmed to a medium heat. I add in the ingredients, add freshly ground pepper, and stir fry to suit.

I like to serve this stir fry with a slice of pepper jack cheddar cheese and garnish it with fresh strawberries

XXI. Sesame Seasoned Long Neck Squash and Red, Yellow Green Bell Pepper and Celery Stir Fry

For this stir fry be sure to add the slices of long neck squash in last: They take very little cooking and – if over-cooked – lose appeal. The bell peppers and celery are much hardier and require more cooking so I introduce them to my Teflon skillet first and – after they are cooked to preference – I add the slices of long neck squash.

During this process I sprinkle in the sesame seeds. For emphasis, the long neck squash slices only need a few minutes in the pan until they are done. As noted before I'm a big fan of freshly ground pepper, so I add this while I stir fry the rest of the ingredients.

We found that this was a wonderful side dish for a fried apple pork sausage picked up fresh from Sunflower Farmer's Market.

Here is a recipe for an Almond Oat Yeast Bread that you can try:

XXII. Almond Oat Yeast Bread

1. Begin with ¼ cup of warm water mixed in a bowl with a teaspoon of sugar and a packet of Hodgson Mills yeast for whole grain flours.

Note: Artificial sweeteners – such as Splenda – can counteract the bacterial action of the yeast. Since these artificial sweeteners tend to be like "mirror images" of real sugar, the yeast will accept them. However, the artificial sweetener does not behave in the same way that sugar does; instead, the artificial sweetener may impede the yeast. You can check the "vitality" of your yeast by waiting a few minutes and observing whether mild "bubbling activity" begins.

2. Thoroughly mix in ½ cup of vital wheat gluten. Set this mixture aside to rise in a warm (but not hot) location for one to two hours.

3. In a separate bowl combine:

- ½ cup of almond flour

- ½ cup of oat flour

- ½ cup of garbanzo flour

- 2 tablespoons of coconut flour

- 1/8 teaspoon of Sea salt

4. Melt 3 tbsp of butter in a Pyrex measuring cup. Blend ¼ cup of unsweetened, unflavoured coconut milk into the butter along with two beaten eggs. You will want to add the coconut milk first to the butter so that the butter – if it is still hot from being melted – does not cook the eggs!

5. Thoroughly mix the butter-eggs-coconut milk mixture into the bowl containing the almond/oat/garbanzo flour to create your non-wheat portion of your bread.

6. Combine the non-wheat portion of your bread with the now raised wheat and yeast portion. The raised wheat and yeast portion will be "elastic" and you will need to work the two mixtures together.

7. The resulting mixture will somewhat resemble a moist, "gritty" cookie dough. Set it aside in a warm (not hot) place and let it rise for several hours.

8. Sprinkle two tablespoons of oat flour and ¼ cup of milled flax seeds over the surface and especially around the sides of the raised mixture.

9. Use a spatula to help pour the raised mixture into a glass loaf pan that has been "greased" with Crisco vegetable shortening.

10. Then bake at 350 degrees for 30 minutes or until done

11. Allow to cool for at least 15 minutes

12. Separate the bread from the sides of the pan with a thin knife

13. Turn the bread out onto a flat surface and allow it to cool.

Slice and serve with butter – it is delicious and only a few net grams of carbs per slice!

XXIII. Fried, Spiced Parmesan and Sesame Seed Diced Tomato with Spinach Dressed Chicken Strips and Bacon

Drizzle an ounce or so of olive oil in a non-stick pan. Arrange the uncooked chicken strips in the pan. Season the chicken with freshly ground pepper, sea salt, and fresh parsley, sage, rosemary and thyme (the Simon and Garfunkel herbs). Sprinkle sesame seeds over the seasoned chicken strips. Liberally spread a mixture of spinach leaves and other fresh salad greens over the chicken. Sprinkle shredded Parmesan cheese over the greens. Position half strips of pre-cooked bacon on the greens (like putting pepperoni on a pizza). Spread one can of low-carb diced tomatoes (read the labels to find the lowest net carb count for your diced tomatoes) over the greens. Add more Parmesan to taste. Cover with either a splatter screen or a piece of non-inked kitchen paper (be careful to

NOT set your kitchen paper on fire!). Then cook for thirty minutes (longer as needed) on a medium to medium-low heat. Check to assure your chicken is thoroughly cooked and that the liquid from your diced tomatoes has simmered down to your preference.

You and your guests will love this AND it is so very easy to prepare!

XXIV. Quick and Delicious Egg Breakfast

Combine a quarter cup of grated cheddar cheese (or some other cheese of your choice) with two or three beaten eggs in a microwavable dish. Add ground pepper and sea salt. Microwave for 90 seconds to 3 minutes depending on your microwave and how firm you like your eggs.

For variety try adding some diced tomatoes, sautéed onions, and diced bell peppers. You could even go "hog" nuts (pardon the pun!) and add some pre-cooked pieces of bacon

XXV. "World War II" Lemonade

Mix one half to one teaspoon of apple cider vinegar with one half to one teaspoon of granulated Stevia with a glass full of iced water. Stir and serve.

Alternately, add some sliced strawberries and some fresh mint leaves.

Why "World War II" lemonade? (No, I was not alive then!)

A grandmother told me that during World War II everything – including lemons – was scarce. On the other hand, vinegar was common and is an excellent substitute for lemon juice.

Of greater concern: Vinegar has virtually no carbs while fruit juices are high carb.

XXVI. Chocolate Craver's Low-Carb Hot Chocolate

Microwave a mug of unsweetened, unflavoured coconut milk until it is just warm. Stir in one to two teaspoons of baker's cocoa with Stevia to taste (normally a teaspoon or less). An overly obvious hint here, but offered anyway: After stirring, lick your spoon to see if your chocolate drink meets your "sweetness" requirements (I sprinkle my Stevia in so there is no concern for contaminated teaspoons if I add more sweetener). Heat the mug of chocolate again in the microwave until hot enough to suit. Garnish with a tablespoon of whipping cream. As you may wish, sprinkle a little baker's cocoa on the whipping cream to dazzle yourself with delicious creativity.

This is low-carb, it is chocolate, and it is a great anytime treat - I especially like a mug before going to bed!

XXVII. Delicious, Low-Carb Fried Chicken

The problem with most fried chicken, chicken nuggets and chicken strips today is the high carb batter that coats it. Here is a delicious way to batter fried chicken and keep your carb count down:

A. You Will Need:

- ½ cup almond flour

- 2 tbsp of milled flax seeds

- 1 tbsp of sesame seeds

- ¼ cup of coconut flour

- ¼ cup granulated Stevia

- 2 tsp of Italian seasoning

- Sea salt and freshly ground pepper to taste (½ tsp – or more – of each)

- 1 egg

- ¼ cup of unsweetened, unflavored coconut milk

- ¼ cup olive oil

- 2 lbs of sectioned chicken pieces (quarters, legs, thighs, breasts – to suit)

- ¼ cup of parsley flakes (fresh if you can get it!)

B. To Prepare:

1. Combine the dry ingredients into a "shaker" bag (a durable, left over plastic grocery bag will work, but I suggest double bagging to avoid spills when you shake the chicken!)

2. Combine and mix the egg and the coconut milk thoroughly in a small, glass pie plate

3. Rinse the chicken pieces under cold water (carefully shaking the excess water off in the sink) and then place the chicken pieces one at a time in the egg and coconut mixture, turning them until they are coated

4. Place each piece one at a time in the shaker bag with the dry ingredients and then shake until coated to your taste (I go light on the coating and find the results are great!)

5. Pour the olive oil into a 10-12 inch Teflon fry pan that has been preheated to a medium-low heat.

6. Place each coated chicken piece into the 10-12 inch Teflon fry pan

7. Sprinkle the parsley onto the chicken

8. Fry the chicken pieces and turn – as needed – until thoroughly cooked. (How long this takes depends on your stove, your pan's heat distributing properties and the thickness of your chicken pieces. For my kitchen, about 15 to 20 minutes per side seems to work.)

9. A splatter guard for your pan is highly recommended. As an alternative, a piece of good kitchen paper (non-inked – ink is not a good food additive!) can be used,

but – of course – caution must be exercised to make certain that the kitchen paper is not set on fire by your stove!

C. This chicken is great for a meal and for in-between meals!

We recently made a batch of this. Not only was it amazing as a main course, but it is a flavourful, healthy, easy in-between meal that stores well in the refrigerator. It can then be eaten cold or warmed up in the microwave.

It sounds so good, I think I will have some now!

XXVIII. Cheese, Onion, Peppers and Bacon Omelet

Here is a great way to add protein to your low-carb eating regimen!

Keep in mind that omelettes are long past the point of being merely a breakfast food: Omelettes are great for lunch, for dinner, and for in-between meals, too.

Though this omelet can take some time to prepare (less time when you are practiced in making it), it is readily prepared in advance and – depending on your appetite – can be portioned into two to four servings.

These omelet portions refrigerate well and are delicious throughout your week: An awesome meal ready to go at the drop of a hat!.

A. You will need

- ¼ green bell pepper
- ¼ red bell pepper
- ½ medium sized sweet onion
- 3 tbsp of butter (we suggest Challenge Butter – creamier more flavourful)
- ¼ cup of unsweetened, unflavored coconut or almond milk
- 2 to 3 strips of precooked bacon
- Sea salt
- black pepper – ready for grinding!
- ¼ to ½ cup of grated cheddar cheese

B. Readying the Omelet Ingredients

1. clean and chop ¼ green pepper and ¼ red pepper

2. remove the outer husk and chop ½ medium sized sweet onion

3. sauté the onion in two tablespoons of butter until beginning to brown

4. stir in and sauté the chopped red and green peppers

5. remove the sautéed vegetables to a separate dish and (if you want your pan to be less sticky when adding the eggs, rinse and dry the pan)

6. melt 1 tbsp of butter in a 10 - 12 inch Teflon pan warmed to a medium low heat

7. beat 4 or 5 eggs (depending on their size and your preference)

8. blend ¼ cup of unsweetened, unflavoured coconut or almond milk into the beaten eggs (I prefer unsweetened, unflavoured coconut milk)

C. Cooking the Omelet

1. Pour the egg and coconut mixture into your pan

2. Season with Sea salt and freshly ground black pepper to taste

3. Distribute ¼ to ½ cup of grated cheddar cheese onto the omelet (other cheeses – such as feta – can readily be substituted and/or the grated cheese could be applied as a topping to the omelet)

4. Allow the omelet to cook for 30 seconds or so

5. Place small portions (each strip of precooked bacon readily tears into 8 to 10 portions) of the pre-cooked bacon around the omelet (like putting pepperoni on a pizza!)

6. Sprinkle the set aside sautéed onions and peppers over the omelet

7. Cook on medium low heat until no longer runny on top.

Alternately, you can cover your pan, but this tends to steam the omelet and makes it rubbery. Accordingly, adjust to your preferences.

(**Note:** This all depends on your pan and your stove temperatures since there is MUCH variability in both. A good pan will distribute the heat evenly. Poor one will require you to move the pan so that runny areas of the cooking omelet receive more heat while the more quickly cooking center section of the omelet is given less heat.)

D. Serving the Omelet

1. A good Teflon pan and pancake turner(s) makes this next part much easier!

2. Choose the firmest edge section of the omelet and use your pancake turner to insure that the edge is separated from the pan.

3. Carefully loosen the bottom of that section's half of the omelet with your pancake turner.

4. Then use the pancake turner (I like to use two pancake turners, one under each quarter of the half omelet that I will "turn") to carefully turn half of the omelet over onto the remaining half.

5. Judging from the bottom portion of the omelet that is now on top, you may want to allow the omelet to cook a bit longer.

Optionally, you can now more easily flip the "halved over" omelet for more cooking of the side that was on top (if you so desire).

6. Turn out the halved omelet onto a serving plate.

7. The halved omelet is easily sectioned into two, three or even four portions (in accordance with your appetite).

E. Saving Portions of the Omelet

Since a small amount of moisture precipitates out of refrigerated omelettes, place each portion that you are saving on a small, microwavable plate onto which you have first placed a plain (no need for ink in your food!) piece of kitchen paper. When you're ready to eat, just microwave the portion already on the plate for about 30 seconds.

Check to see if it is warm enough. Another 20 seconds should be sufficient if you like it piping hot. Do NOT overheat in your microwave or your omelet will become rubbery!

XXIX. Almond Flour Cranberry (or, Blueberry) Loaf

A. You will need:

- 2 cups of almond flour

- ¼ cup of milled flax seeds

- 1/8 cup of sesame seeds

- ½ cup of granulated Stevia

- 2 tbsp of baking soda (make sure it is fresh and active!)

- 1 tsp of apple cider vinegar

- 1/8 tsp of salt (we like Sea salt)

- 4 tsp of pumpkin pie spice (vary this to suit your taste)

- 1 tsp of nutmeg

- 2 fresh eggs, beaten

- ¼ cup of unsweetened, unflavored coconut milk (we are at high altitude - adjust your fluid in this mixture as needed)

- ¼ cup of olive oil

- ¼ to ½ cup fresh or frozen cranberries or blueberries (to suit your taste)

- Butter to coat the inside of your Pyrex loaf pan

B. Preparation

1. Preheat your oven to 350 degrees

2. Combine your dry ingredients in a sufficiently large bowl and then stir in the teaspoon of apple cider vinegar

3. Mix the eggs, coconut milk and olive oil in a separate bowl

4. Add and mix the wet and dry ingredients

5. Blend in the fresh or frozen fruit (cranberries or blueberries)

6. Place in a buttered, medium sized Pyrex loaf pan

7. Let the preparation sit for 15 minutes

8. Bake at 350 degrees for 30 to 40 minutes (the sides of the loaf will begin to brown and an inserted toothpick will come out dry)

9. Let the baked loaf sit for an hour

10. Run a thin knife around the sides of the baked loaf to separate it from the Pyrex pan

11. Carefully turn the loaf out onto a flat surface

12. Let the loaf cool for at least one hour. Slice and serve with butter!

This bread is a work in process: Please experiment and let me know what you find. Also, though I find the flavour and texture of this bread acceptable, you may not! Please allow for personal preference and – again – keep in mind that this "bread" is not at all like store bought sandwich breads. If anything, it is more like a coarse, banana loaf.

Note: This is a loaf that tastes better after it has sat (covered, please – we don't want it to dry out too much!) for one full day, though it can be eaten within a few hours of baking.

XXX. Split Chicken Breast Served with buttered and sautéed asparagus

*This is easiest if you already have a bunch of this stuff on hand!

. . . I only had to get the chicken . . .

A. You will need:

- A package of generous sized chicken breasts

(I got three breasts in a package from Safeway at $1.99/lb) – it came to $4.53

- Butter (Challenge Butter is better and on sale was $1.99/lb)

- Olive Oil (At the time: $6.99 for 32 ounces at Sunflower Market)

*In my recent experience, the price of olive oil has roughly doubled since Sprouts replaced the Sunflower Market where I shop.

- Marinara sauce or diced tomatoes. Safeway has a house brand

*It is possible to fine "Organic Basil" Marinara sauce with 6 grams of net carb per serving (8 grams of carb less 2 grams of fiber).

On the other hand, if you read labels carefully, it is possible to get a can of diced tomatoes in the 2 to 3 net grams of carbs per serving range.

- Six slices of bacon

- A fresh "stand" of asparagus (rubber banded together at Walmart for a couple of dollars)

- Fresh spinach leaves

- Salt (we like Sea Salt) and pepper (we prefer freshly ground)

- Italian seasonings (lots of options here – fresh is better)

- Sesame Seeds (a small container from the spice aisle)

- Milled Flax Seed (check Whole Foods or Sunflower Market)

- A few ounces of unsweetened coconut or almond milk

- Cheddar Cheese for grating (I like Sharp or Extra Sharp)

- Grated parmesan and Romano cheese (comes in a shaker – fresh is nice!)

B. Chicken Preparation

1. Cut the chicken breast in half lengthwise (making two portions of each breast).

a) Then cut each breast almost entirely in half sideways (this filets the chicken breast portions so each is half as thick but now lays out flat to cover twice as much area)

b) Lay the filleted chicken breasts in a flat, glass cooking dish that has been lightly coated in olive oil.

2. Season the chicken breast filets with Sea Salt, freshly ground pepper, and Italian Seasoning (to taste – I like to be generous!).

3. Liberally sprinkle sesame seeds on each seasoned filet.

4. Place liberal quantities of fresh spinach on each open faced filet.

5. Place a strip of bacon on top of the spinach.

6. Garnish the bacon/spinach with marinara sauce or diced tomatoes (richer flavour comes from good marinara, but the diced tomatoes can be easier and lower carb).

7. Liberally (the flavour is in the fat!) sprinkle the parmesan Romano cheese on each garnished fillet.

8. Pour a small quantity (a few tablespoons, depending on the size of your baking dish) of water between each filet (do NOT submerge the filets!). Our goal here is keep our chicken moist while it bake (the bacon aids in this) and to create uniformity in baking.

9. Bake in a preheated oven at 325 degrees until done (45 to 60 minutes).

Serve fresh from the oven with the buttered and cheddar cheese sautéed asparagus (see next page for the asparagus and sauce)!

This will serve six (who will want more!).

C. Asparagus Preparation

1. Clean the asparagus by running it under cold water.

2. Cut and discard the bottom few inches of the base of the asparagus so that only the tender, non-woody portions of the asparagus remain.

3. Place the asparagus in the bottom of a 10 inch Teflon frying pan that has been coated with about one eighth to one quarter inch of warmed water (warm the water by heating on the stove at medium to medium low heat – CO Springs is high altitude, so adjust as needed).

4. Cook the asparagus until tender (about ten minutes).

5. Remove the asparagus to a serving dish.

6. Coat the asparagus in challenge butter.

7. Prepare the cheddar cheese asparagus sauté:

a) warm a saucepan to medium low

b) melt a few tablespoons of Challenge Butter in a sauté pan

c) stir in a few ounces of milk (almond or coconut milk, if you like)

d) stir in a few tablespoons of Milled Flax Seed

e) grate in and stir a half cup (or more!) of cheddar cheese

f) ready when warm and blended: garnish the asparagus!

*I served this with lime infused water and an easy dessert of King Soopers Carb Control Vanilla Flavoured Yogurt (low cost, low-carb and delicious!) garnished with freshly sliced strawberries.

**The entire meal took me a half hour of actual food preparation AND it was a knockout in flavour and nutrition!

XXXI. Low-Carb Strata

Note: A strata is a layered, crust less quiche.

A. Preheat your oven to 425 degrees:

- Place 3 tablespoons of butter in a deep dish Pyrex pie pan
- Put the dish and butter in the oven for just long enough to melt the butter
- Remove the pan from the oven

B. In a mixing bowl combine:

- 6 beaten eggs
- 1/2 cup of CarbQuik flour

- 1/8 teaspoon salt

- 1/2 cup of unsweetened, unflavored coconut milk

C. Sauté in butter:

- 1/4 diced sweet onion

- 1/2 cup of diced fresh or frozen broccoli

- 1/2 cup of diced celery

- allow this to cool for a few minutes before combining with the egg mixture

D. Pour half of the egg mixture into the pie pan:

- add in the sautéed onion/broccoli/celery

- liberally sprinkle grated cheddar cheese and/or Parmesan over the mixture now combined with the sautéed vegetables

- season with ground pepper and sea salt to suit

- arrange chunks of bacon over the mixture (like putting pepperoni on a pizza)

- pour the other half of the egg mixture over this first layer

- garnish with more grated choose and herbs (parsley, chives, rosemary, sage) to suit

E. Bake at 425 degrees for about 30 minutes:

The strata will develop a beautiful, golden brown top.

Allow it to cool to a comfortable eating temperature and then serve with sliced strawberries and low-carb sour cream!

XXXII. Low-Carb Pancakes

Note: These are really intended for Step Five: Maintaining Our Low-Carb Lifestyle For A Lifetime. Even though CarbQuik is high fiber and low-carb, eating it may stimulate carb craving.

A. Create Your Pancake Batter:

- Add a beaten egg to your mixing bowl

- Mix in 3/4 cup of CarbQuik flour

- Combine this mixture with 1/4 teaspoon of salt and 1 tablespoon of granulated Stevia

- Optionally, add in a tablespoon of cinnamon (I recommend this!)

- Mix in about 1/2 cup of unsweetened, unflavored coconut milk (more or less depending on how thick you like your pancakes)

B. Melt Two Tablespoons Of Butter In A Teflon Pan Set At A Medium Heat:

- allow for this spreading as you pour the batter)–Pour in small quantities of pancake batter (the CarbQuik makes the batter spread more than traditional flour

- Allow the pancakes to cook properly before attempting to turn them

- You'll have to be careful in turning the pancakes (they crumble easily)

C. Serve With Your Choice Of Eggs, Meats, Melons and Berries!

- I like to top mine with butter and with low-carb syrups (yep, they exist!)

- These pancakes are so good, we sometimes use them as a side with lunch or dinner!

XXXIII. Peanut Butter and Bacon Breakfast Soft Taco

Note: This recipe is a favourite for my wife. In addition to the basic ingredients, she sometimes adds homemade coconut butter and/or slices of avocado.

Heat your bacon

- 2 strips of bacon per tortilla

- Spread chunky peanut butter on a Mission Carb Control Small Fajita tortilla

- Arrange the heated bacon on the peanut buttered low-car tortilla

- Fold over and enjoy!

XXXIV. Homemade Coconut Butter

Note: This recipe is a favourite for my wife. Be sure to use unsweetened coconut flakes.

Prepare to blend!

- Add a portion of the contents of a 1 pound bag of unsweetened coconut flakes into your blender

- Puree and/or pulse and continue adding coconut flakes from the bag

- Periodically scrape the blender container with a spatula in order to ensure thorough blending

- When blended to suit, scrape the contents into a storage container

- As explained above, this is a nice addition to the Peanut Butter and Bacon Breakfast Soft Taco!

In addition, the Coconut Butter can be a flavourful and nutritious addition to hot chocolate or hot coffee!

www.ingramcontent.com/pod-product-compliance
Lightning Source LLC
Chambersburg PA
CBHW070631290526

45790CB00001B/76